Your KIDNEYS, Your Way

PERSONALIZED STRATEGIES

FOR

LIVING WELL WITH CKD

(CHRONIC KIDNEY DISEASE)

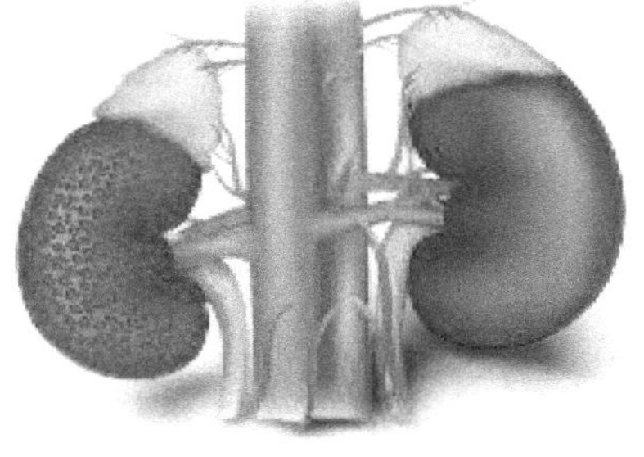

BY: DR. JADEN CLINTON

COPYRIGHT©JADENCLINTON

This book is intended for educational and informational purposes only. The content presented within is meant to contribute to the understanding and appreciation of the subject matter, health matters. Any references to specific events, names, or copyrighted material are used for the purpose of commentary, criticism, or review.

The author and publisher disclaim responsibility for any adverse effects resulting directly or indirectly from information contained in this book.

TABLE OF CONTENT

INTRODUCTION

Virtualize this: Jessica, a vibrant 38-year-old yoga instructor, had been feeling unusually tired for weeks. She dismissed it as just a result of her busy schedule. But a routine blood test brought a startling revelation: she had chronic kidney disease (CKD). Suddenly, her life of yoga mats and laughter felt distant and uncertain.

However, Jessica's story is one of resilience and transformation. Equipped with knowledge and a proactive mindset, she revamped her lifestyle. She educated herself on dietary management, discovered the benefits of CKD-specific exercise, and found support in a caring community. Today, Jessica is not only managing her condition but thriving. Through her social media platform, "Living Loud with CKD," she inspires countless others.

Jessica's experience is far from unique. Millions of people live with CKD, a condition that affects kidney function. It can be daunting, but here's the empowering truth: you have the ability to significantly improve your well-being with CKD.

This book, Your Kidneys, Your Way, is not a generic guide. It's a personalized roadmap to managing CKD. We'll dive into real-life stories, like Jessica's. We'll also meet John, a 65-year-old grandfather who rediscovered joy in gardening after his CKD diagnosis. And Sarah, a young professional who built a successful career while managing her condition.

Through these stories, you'll learn about:

- The varied symptoms of CKD, from fatigue to high blood pressure.
- Simple yet effective dietary changes that can make a big difference.
- Exercise routines tailored for those with CKD, from gentle walks to strength training.
- The importance of managing stress and building a supportive network for emotional health.
- The latest advancements in CKD research and treatment options.

This book aims to empower you to take charge of your health journey. It offers practical tools, dispels common myths, and celebrates the successes of those living well with CKD. You'll learn how to:

- Collaborate with your healthcare team to develop a personalized action plan.
- Make informed decisions about your diet and exercise regimen.
- Advocate for yourself and navigate the healthcare system confidently.
- Foster a positive mindset and cultivate a lifestyle that suits your unique needs.

CKD may be a part of your life, but it doesn't have to define it. With the right knowledge, actions, and personalized approach, you can thrive. Take a deep breath, turn the page, and start your empowering journey to living well with CKD.

CHAPTER ONE

THE KIDNEY POWERHOUSE: UNVEILING THE VITAL ROLE OF YOUR KIDNEYS

1.1 BEYOND FILTRATION: THE SYMPHONY OF KIDNEY FUNCTIONS

Imagine your kidneys as a state-of-the-art water treatment plant, meticulously filtering and purifying your blood. But that's just the beginning of their incredible performance. These bean-shaped organs are like the conductors of a grand orchestra, harmonizing a symphony of essential functions that keep you healthy and thriving. Let's go deeper into their talents.

1. Waste Disposal: The Dirty Job, Done Right

Your kidneys are tireless filtration units, constantly sifting through your blood to remove waste products generated by your body's activities. Every cell produces byproducts like ammonia and urea, which can be toxic if they accumulate. Your kidneys expertly identify and remove these wastes, sending them out with your urine.

But waste disposal isn't a one-size-fits-all job. Your kidneys act as discerning garbage collectors, meticulously sorting through the blood. They hold onto essential nutrients and electrolytes, such as sodium, potassium, and calcium, which your body needs. They then precisely adjust the concentration of these elements in your blood, maintaining a delicate balance crucial for muscle function, nerve impulses, and overall health.

2. Blood Pressure Regulation: Keeping the Flow Just Right

Think of your blood pressure as the water pressure in your house. It needs to be strong enough to deliver blood to all your organs but not so high that it damages your blood vessels. Your kidneys play a key role in maintaining this balance. They produce a hormone called renin, which triggers a cascade of events leading to the relaxation of blood vessels, thus lowering blood pressure. Additionally, they help regulate the amount of fluid in your body—too much fluid can raise blood pressure, while dehydration can cause it to drop. By managing fluid volume, your kidneys significantly contribute to maintaining a healthy blood pressure range.

3. Red Blood Cell Production: The Symphony Needs Its Players

Red blood cells are essential for carrying oxygen throughout your body, but they don't last forever, and your body needs a constant supply. This is where your kidneys step in with another surprising act—they produce a hormone called erythropoietin (EPO), which stimulates your bone marrow to produce red blood cells, ensuring a continual flow of oxygen to your tissues.

4. Bone Health: A Supporting Role

Strong bones are crucial for supporting your body and protecting your organs. Your kidneys play a behind-the-scenes role in maintaining bone health by producing an active form of vitamin D. This vitamin D helps your body absorb calcium from your diet, which is essential for building and maintaining strong bones.

5. Acid-Base Balance: Maintaining the Perfect Harmony

Your body's pH level, a measure of acidity or alkalinity, needs to be tightly controlled for optimal function. Just like a well-tuned orchestra needs all instruments in perfect harmony, your bodily processes generate acidic byproducts that need to be balanced. Your kidneys act as a buffer, neutralizing these acids and maintaining a healthy pH level in your blood.

Your kidneys are far more than just filtration units. They are a complex and vital organ system orchestrating a symphony of functions that keep you healthy. Understanding the diverse roles your kidneys play can empower you to take charge of your health and appreciate the incredible work they do every minute of the day.

1.2 The Silent Threat: Understanding Chronic Kidney Disease (CKD)

Chronic Kidney Disease (CKD)—just hearing the name can be intimidating. It might bring to mind images of dialysis machines and restrictions. But knowledge is power. Understanding CKD is the first step towards taking control of your health and leading a fulfilling life.

A Slow and Stealthy Thief

Unlike sudden illnesses, CKD often creeps in gradually, like a slow, silent thief. In its early stages, CKD may not show any noticeable symptoms. You might feel completely fine, going about your daily life, while your kidneys are slowly losing their ability to function properly. This is why CKD is often referred to as a "silent threat."

The Culprits Behind the Curtain

Several underlying conditions can lead to CKD. High blood pressure and diabetes are two of the most common causes. When these conditions are not well-managed, they can damage the delicate filtering units in your kidneys, leading to a gradual decline in their function.

Other risk factors for CKD include

- A family history of kidney disease
- Certain autoimmune diseases
- Polycystic Kidney Disease (PKD), a genetic condition that causes cysts to grow on the kidneys
- Recurrent urinary tract infections (UTIs)
- Long-term use of certain medications

Losing the Rhythm: How CKD Affects Your Body

As CKD progresses, your kidneys become less efficient at their jobs, leading to a buildup of waste products in your blood. Imagine your body's filtration system getting clogged, causing toxins to accumulate instead of being eliminated. This disrupts the delicate balance your kidneys maintain within your body.

Here's how CKD can impact some of the vital functions discussed in Chapter 1.1

Waste Disposal: With reduced filtration capacity, waste products may not be effectively removed from your blood, leading to fatigue, nausea, and difficulty concentrating.

Blood Pressure Regulation: CKD can impair your kidneys' ability to regulate blood pressure, increasing the risk of heart disease and stroke.

Red Blood Cell Production: Reduced EPO production due to CKD can lead to anemia, causing fatigue, shortness of breath, and pale skin.

Bone Health: Impaired vitamin D activation due to CKD can weaken bones, increasing the risk of fractures.

Acid-Base Balance: CKD can compromise your kidneys' ability to regulate blood pH, leading to acidosis, which can cause fatigue, nausea, and bone problems.

The Importance of Early Detection

The good news is that CKD is often treatable, especially when detected early. By identifying CKD in its early stages, you can take steps to slow its progression and manage the associated risks. Regular checkups with your doctor, including blood and urine tests, are crucial for early detection.

Living Well with CKD: Taking Control of Your Journey

A CKD diagnosis doesn't have to be a life sentence. With proper management and a proactive approach, you can live a full and healthy life. This book is your guide on that journey. We'll explore strategies for managing your diet, exercise routines tailored for CKD, and the importance of building a strong support system. You'll learn about treatment options and how to work effectively with your healthcare team. Most importantly, you'll discover how to embrace a positive mindset and live well with CKD.

Recall, knowledge is power. By understanding CKD and taking charge of your health, you can quiet the "silent threat" and keep your body's symphony playing in perfect harmony.

1.3 Stages of CKD: A Roadmap for Your Journey

Imagine a long road trip across breathtaking landscapes. Just like any journey, CKD has different stages, each with its unique terrain. Understanding these stages can help you navigate your CKD journey with confidence, allowing you to set realistic goals, tailor your approach, and celebrate milestones along the way.

The Roadmap Revealed: Stages of CKD

CKD is classified into five stages based on the estimated Glomerular Filtration Rate (eGFR), a measure of how well your kidneys filter waste products from your blood. Here's a breakdown of each stage:

Stage 1: Early CKD (eGFR > 90 ml/min/1.73 m²)

In this earliest stage, you might not experience any symptoms, but your eGFR indicates a slight decrease in kidney function. This is a wake-up call to take action and implement healthy lifestyle changes to slow down further decline.

Stage 2: Mild CKD (eGFR 60-89 ml/min/1.73 m²)

Similar to Stage 1, you may not notice any symptoms. However, the decrease in eGFR is more significant. This is a crucial time to work with your doctor to develop a personalized management plan, which may include dietary changes, blood pressure control, and regular monitoring of kidney function.

Stage 3: Moderate CKD (eGFR 30-59 ml/min/1.73 m²)

Stage 3 is divided into 3a (eGFR 45-59 ml/min/1.73 m²) and 3b (eGFR 30-44 ml/min/1.73 m²). As your eGFR declines, you might start experiencing symptoms like fatigue, high blood pressure, or difficulty concentrating. This stage emphasizes strict management of your diet, medications, and risk factors like diabetes and high blood pressure.

Stage 4: Severe CKD (eGFR 15-29 ml/min/1.73 m²)

At this stage, your kidney function is significantly reduced. Waste products may start accumulating in your blood, leading to more noticeable symptoms like fatigue, nausea, and difficulty sleeping. This stage often involves working with a nephrologist (a kidney specialist) to explore treatment options like dialysis or kidney transplantation.

Stage 5: End-Stage Renal Disease (ESRD) (eGFR < 15 ml/min/1.73 m² or dialysis)

This is the most advanced stage of CKD, where your kidneys can no longer function on their own to meet your body's needs. Dialysis, a process that removes waste products from your blood, or a kidney transplant becomes necessary to maintain your health.

Beyond the Numbers: A Personalized Approach

While the eGFR is a valuable tool for staging CKD, it's just one piece of the puzzle. Your doctor will consider your overall health, symptoms, and risk factors to determine the best course of action for you. There's no one-size-fits-all approach to CKD management.

A Roadmap, not a Destination

Think of the stages of CKD as a roadmap, not a final destination. By understanding these stages and working proactively with your healthcare team, you can take control of your journey. Early detection and treatment can significantly impact your prognosis. This book will equip you with strategies for each stage, empowering you to slow down the progression of CKD and live a fulfilling life.

Every milestone, every step towards a healthier lifestyle, is a victory on your CKD journey. This book is your guide, cheering you on every mile of the way!

CHAPTER TWO

RECOGNIZING THE SIGNS: EARLY DETECTION AND DIAGNOSIS OF CKD

2.1 DON'T IGNORE THE CLUES: COMMON SYMPTOMS OF CKD

Chronic Kidney Disease (CKD) can be a sneaky culprit, often developing gradually without noticeable symptoms in the early stages. This can make it easy to dismiss subtle signs, especially when we're busy with our daily lives. However, your body has ways of communicating, even in whispers. Here, we'll explore some common symptoms of CKD that you shouldn't ignore.

Feeling Fatigued All the Time?

One of the most common complaints among people with CKD is fatigue. You might feel constantly drained, lacking the energy you once had for even simple tasks. This can be caused by a buildup of waste products in your blood, which can make your body work harder to function.

Frequent Urination, Day and Night

Changes in your bathroom habits can be a red flag for CKD. You might find yourself needing to urinate more often, even during the night. This could be due to your kidneys struggling to properly concentrate urine, leading to increased production of diluted urine.

Blood in Your Urine (Hematuria)

Seeing blood in your urine can be alarming, but it's important to stay calm and consult your doctor. Blood in your urine can sometimes be a sign of CKD, but it can also have other causes. Early detection and diagnosis are key.

Puffy Eyes and Swollen Ankles: Fluid Retention Issues

As your kidneys lose their filtering ability, excess fluid can build up in your body. This can manifest as puffiness around your eyes, swelling in your ankles, or even general edema (fluid retention) throughout your body.

Loss of Appetite and Metallic Taste

Changes in taste and appetite can occur with CKD. You might experience a metallic taste in your mouth, leading to a decreased desire to eat. This can be caused by a buildup of waste products and hormonal imbalances associated with CKD.

Itchy Skin and Dryness

Healthy skin relies on proper waste removal and balanced fluid levels. CKD can disrupt these processes, leading to dry, itchy skin.

Trouble Sleeping and Difficulty Concentrating

The disrupted sleep you experience with CKD can be a vicious cycle. The fatigue and difficulty concentrating can further impact your sleep quality. This domino effect can significantly affect your daily life.

High Blood Pressure (Hypertension)

High blood pressure is both a risk factor for and a symptom of CKD. When your kidneys aren't functioning optimally, it can lead to difficulty regulating blood pressure. It's crucial to monitor your blood pressure regularly and work with your doctor to keep it under control.

Not All Symptoms Mean CKD

It's important to remember that these symptoms can also be caused by other conditions. However, if you're experiencing several of them, it's best to consult your doctor for a thorough evaluation. Early detection of CKD is crucial for managing its progression and improving your long-term health.

Beyond the List: Listening to Your Body

This list provides a starting point, but don't underestimate the power of your own intuition. You know your body best. If you're experiencing any changes in how you feel, even if they seem subtle, it's worth talking to your doctor.

Early Intervention is Key

The good news is that by catching CKD early and adopting a proactive approach, you can significantly impact its progression and manage the associated symptoms.

2.2 Blood Tests and Beyond: Tools for Early Detection

Imagine Chronic Kidney Disease (CKD) as a puzzle. Early detection is like finding the corner pieces—it sets the stage for putting the whole picture together and taking control of your health journey. In this chapter, we'll explore the valuable tools your doctor can use to detect CKD in its early stages, even before you experience any symptoms.

The Blood Test Detectives: Unveiling Clues

Blood tests are the first line of defense in detecting CKD. These simple tests can provide valuable clues about how well your kidneys are functioning. Here's a breakdown of some key blood tests used for CKD detection:

- Glomerular Filtration Rate (GFR): This measures how well your kidneys are filtering waste products from your blood. A lower-than-normal eGFR can indicate CKD.

- Blood Urea Nitrogen (BUN) and Creatinine: These are waste products normally removed from your blood by your kidneys. Elevated levels can suggest impaired kidney function.

- Electrolytes: Your kidneys help maintain the balance of electrolytes like potassium, sodium, and calcium in your blood. Abnormal levels can be a red flag for CKD.

Urinalysis: Unveiling the Story in Your Urine

A urinalysis is another simple test that can provide valuable information about your kidney health. It analyzes your urine for abnormalities like

Protein: Healthy kidneys don't allow large amounts of protein to pass into your urine. The presence of protein can be a sign of kidney damage.

Blood: The presence of blood cells in your urine can warrant further investigation.

Unusual Cells: Abnormal cells in your urine may signal inflammation or other issues in your urinary tract, potentially linked to CKD.

Imaging Techniques: Seeing is Believing

Sometimes, your doctor may recommend imaging tests to get a clearer picture of your kidneys. These tests can help identify any abnormalities in their size or structure that might be contributing to CKD. Common imaging techniques include:

Ultrasound: This painless test uses sound waves to create an image of your kidneys.

CT scan or MRI: These scans provide detailed cross-sectional images of your kidneys, allowing for a more comprehensive evaluation.

24-Hour Urine Collection: A Day in the Life of Your Kidneys

This test involves collecting all your urine over a 24-hour period. It allows your doctor to measure the total amount of waste products and electrolytes eliminated by your kidneys.

Don't Be Afraid to Ask Questions

These are just some of the tools available for detecting CKD. It's important to communicate openly with your doctor about your risk factors and any concerns you may have. Don't hesitate to ask questions like:

- What tests do you recommend for me?
- What do the results of my tests mean?
- How often should I be screened for CKD?
- Early Detection is Empowering

Early detection of CKD allows you and your doctor to take action early. By adopting a healthy lifestyle, managing risk factors like high blood pressure and diabetes, and potentially starting treatment, if necessary, you can significantly impact the progression of CKD and improve your long-term health.

Think of these tests as proactive measures, empowering you to take charge of your health and maintain optimal kidney function for years to come.

2.3 The Doctor is in: Understanding Diagnosis and Next Steps

Receiving a diagnosis of chronic kidney disease (CKD) can feel overwhelming. You might have many questions and concerns, but remember, knowledge is power. This chapter will help you understand your diagnosis, what it means for you, and the next steps on your CKD journey.

Understanding Your Diagnosis

Your doctor will explain your diagnosis based on your test results and how well your kidneys are functioning. They might use terms like "stage" or "GFR" to describe the severity of your CKD. Refer back to Chapter 1.3 for a refresher on the stages of CKD and their significance.

Identifying the Cause of Your CKD

Once diagnosed, your doctor will work to determine the underlying cause of your CKD. Here are some common causes:

High Blood Pressure and Diabetes: These conditions can damage the delicate filtering units in your kidneys, leading to CKD.

Autoimmune Diseases: Certain autoimmune diseases can attack the kidneys, causing inflammation and impairing their function.

Polycystic Kidney Disease (PKD): This genetic condition causes cysts to grow on the kidneys, affecting their ability to function properly.

Recurrent Urinary Tract Infections (UTIs): Repeated UTIs can increase the risk of kidney damage if left untreated.

Long-Term Medication Use: Some medications, if taken for a long time, can negatively impact kidney function.

Knowing the cause of your CKD allows your doctor to tailor a treatment plan specifically for you.

Building Your Healthcare Support System

A CKD diagnosis doesn't mean you have to face it alone. You'll work with a team of healthcare professionals to manage your condition and improve your well-being. Here are some key members of your CKD care team:

Nephrologist: A kidney specialist who will provide expert guidance on managing your CKD and coordinate your overall treatment plan.

Primary Care Physician: Your regular doctor who will oversee your general health and work with your nephrologist.

Dietitian: A registered dietitian will create a personalized diet plan to support your kidney health and manage conditions like high blood pressure or diabetes.

Nurse: Your nurse will answer questions, provide education about CKD, and monitor your progress.

Pharmacist: Your pharmacist will ensure you understand your medications, answer any questions, and monitor for potential side effects.

Next Steps for Managing Your CKD

After your diagnosis and understanding the cause of your CKD, your doctor will discuss your treatment plan. Here are some possible components:

Lifestyle Modifications: These form the foundation of CKD management. Changes may include dietary adjustments, exercise recommendations, and smoking cessation to improve overall health and support kidney function.

Medications: Your doctor may prescribe medications to manage blood pressure, control blood sugar levels (if you have diabetes), treat anemia associated with CKD, and reduce waste products in your blood.

Monitoring and Follow-Up: Regular checkups and monitoring your kidney function through blood and urine tests are crucial for tracking progress and adjusting your treatment plan as needed.

Open Communication is Key

Throughout your CKD journey, keep communication lines open with your healthcare team. Ask questions, voice concerns, and discuss any challenges you face in managing your condition. Remember, they are your partners in optimizing your health and well-being.

Building a Strong Support System

Your support system extends beyond medical professionals. Surround yourself with friends, family, and support groups who can offer emotional support and encouragement on your CKD journey. The next chapter will explore strategies for building a strong and supportive network.

CHAPTER THREE

YOUR CKD TEAM: BUILDING A STRONG SUPPORT SYSTEM

3.1 THE POWER OF PARTNERSHIP: WORKING WITH YOUR NEPHROLOGIST

A diagnosis of CKD can bring a wave of emotions—uncertainty, fear, maybe even a bit of confusion. But amidst all that, there's a bright spot: your nephrologist. This kidney specialist becomes your partner in navigating the CKD journey, empowering you to take charge of your health.

Your Kidney Champion: What a Nephrologist Does

Think of your nephrologist as your personal champion for kidney health. They have a deep understanding of CKD, its complexities, and the latest treatment options. Here's what your nephrologist can do for you:

Diagnosis and Treatment Plan: They'll analyze your test results, identify the root cause of your CKD, and create a personalized treatment plan tailored to your specific needs and stage of CKD.

Medication Management: Your nephrologist will prescribe medications to manage your CKD and associated conditions like high blood pressure or diabetes. They'll monitor your medication regimen and adjust it as needed to ensure optimal results with minimal side effects.

Monitoring and Follow-up: Regular checkups with your nephrologist are crucial for tracking your progress. They'll monitor your kidney function through blood and urine tests, check your blood pressure, and assess your overall well-being.

Education and Support: They'll educate you about CKD, its progression, and the importance of lifestyle modifications. They'll answer your questions, address your concerns, and empower you to make informed decisions about your health.

Building a Strong Doctor-Patient Relationship

An effective partnership with your nephrologist requires open communication and trust. Here are some tips to build a strong doctor-patient relationship:

Come Prepared: Before your appointments, jot down any questions, concerns, or changes you've noticed in your health.

Be Clear and Concise: Clearly articulate your symptoms, questions, and any challenges you're facing with treatment.

Speak Up and Advocate for Yourself: Don't hesitate to express your preferences and concerns about your treatment plan.

Bring a Support Person: Consider having a family member or friend accompany you to appointments—they can take notes and offer additional support.

Actively Participate in Your Care: Ask questions, clarify any information you don't understand, and take steps to implement your treatment plan at home.

Beyond the Appointment: Communication is Key

Remember, communication isn't a one-way street. Don't wait until your next appointment to reach out. If you have questions, concerns, or new symptoms between visits, contact your nephrologist's office. They might schedule you for an unscheduled visit or address your concerns over the phone.

Working Together for Your Well-being

Your nephrologist is your trusted advisor and partner in managing CKD. By building a strong relationship based on open communication, you empower yourself to take charge of your health and navigate the path toward a fulfilling life with CKD.

3.2 Beyond the Doctor: The Role of Nurses, Dietitians, and Social Workers

Your nephrologist plays a crucial role in managing your CKD, but they are just one part of your healthcare dream team. Nurses, dietitians, and social workers also play vital roles in supporting your well-being and empowering you throughout your CKD journey.

The Navigators: Nurses Guiding Your Care

Nurses are the backbone of any healthcare team and your constant companions on the CKD journey. Here's how they contribute to your care:

Patient Education: Nurses provide invaluable education about CKD, treatment options, and self-care techniques. They can explain medications, answer your questions clearly, and address any anxieties you might have.

Monitoring and Support: During appointments, nurses take your vital signs, measure your weight, and monitor other key parameters. They also offer emotional support and a listening ear.

Procedural Support: Nurses assist with procedures like blood draws or administering medications.

Treatment Management: They teach you about dialysis (if needed) and other treatment modalities, answering any questions you have about the process.

Advocacy and Coordination: Nurses advocate for your needs and ensure smooth communication between you, your doctor, and other healthcare professionals.

The Food Whisperers: Dietitians Optimizing Your Diet

Nutrition plays a critical role in managing CKD, and this is where your dietitian steps in. They act as your personal food whisperer, guiding you towards a kidney-friendly diet. Here's how they help:

Personalized Meal Plan: They create a customized meal plan based on your stage of CKD, nutritional needs, and preferences. This plan helps you manage blood pressure, control blood sugar (if you have diabetes), and limit waste products your kidneys struggle to filter.

Dietary Education: They educate you about the importance of specific nutrients for kidney health and how to make healthy choices.

Grocery Shopping Guidance: They offer tips on navigating the grocery store, choosing the right foods, and understanding food labels.

Cooking Skills and Recipes: Your dietitian provides delicious recipes and tips for cooking healthy, flavorful meals that fit your needs.

Problem-Solving and Support: They help you navigate challenges like managing food cravings, dining out, or overcoming limitations due to your condition.

The Emotional Anchors: Social Workers Addressing Your Well-being

CKD can significantly impact your emotional well-being. Social workers act as your emotional anchors, providing invaluable support. Here's how they contribute to your care:

Emotional Support and Counseling: They offer individual or group counseling sessions to help you cope with the emotional challenges of living with CKD, including anxiety, depression, or fear of the future.

Social Support Network Building: They help you connect with support groups or resources that provide emotional and social support from others living with CKD.

Financial Assistance: Social workers assist in navigating healthcare costs and exploring financial assistance options if needed.

Social and Practical Issues: They help with challenges like transportation to appointments, meal preparation, or finding help with household chores if your CKD makes daily activities difficult.

Advocacy and Rights Information: They educate you about your rights as a patient and advocate for your needs within the healthcare system.

A Team Approach to Your Well-being

Your nephrologist, nurses, dietitians, and social workers work together as a cohesive team, each contributing their expertise to your overall well-being. Don't hesitate to reach out to any member of your team if you have questions, concerns, or need support. By collaborating with your healthcare dream team, you can effectively manage your CKD and live a fulfilling life.

3.3 Building Your Support Network: Family, Friends, and Community Resources

Living with CKD can sometimes feel isolating, but you don't have to go through it alone. Surrounding yourself with a strong support network of loved ones and tapping into community resources can significantly enhance your well-being.

The Pillars of Support: Family and Friends

Your closest family and friends are often your biggest cheerleaders. Here's how they can be a valuable part of your support system:

Emotional Support: They can be a listening ear, a shoulder to cry on, and a source of encouragement. Sharing your concerns and challenges with loved ones who care about you can be a powerful way to manage stress and anxiety.

Practical Help: Whether it's help with grocery shopping, cooking meals, or transportation to appointments, your loved ones can offer practical assistance that can ease the burden of managing CKD.

Social Connection: They can help you stay socially connected, especially if CKD makes it difficult to participate in activities you once enjoyed. Plan outings, invite them over for board games, or simply have regular phone calls to maintain social interaction.

Advocacy: Sometimes, it can be helpful to have someone accompany you to appointments or speak up on your behalf. Your loved ones can be your advocates, ensuring your needs and concerns are heard.

Communicating with Your Loved Ones

Open communication is key to building a strong support network. Here are some tips for effectively communicating with your family and friends about your CKD:

Explain Your Diagnosis: Briefly explain what CKD is, how it affects you, and any limitations you might have.

Let Them Know Your Needs: Be clear about the kind of support you need, whether it's emotional support, practical help, or simply a listening ear.

Address Their Concerns: They might have questions or anxieties about your condition. Be patient, answer their questions honestly, and address any misconceptions they might have.

Express Your Appreciation: Don't take their support for granted. Thank them for being there for you and express how much their presence means to you.

Strength in Numbers: Support Groups and Community Resources

Beyond your loved ones, there's a broader support system waiting to be tapped into. Here are some valuable resources that can offer support and guidance:

Support Groups: Connecting with others living with CKD can be incredibly empowering. Support groups provide a safe space to share experiences, learn from each other, and find strength in knowing you're not alone. Look for online or in-person support groups in your area.

Kidney Organizations: National and local kidney organizations offer a wealth of information, resources, and support programs. They can connect you with support groups, educational materials, and advocacy initiatives.

Online Communities: Online forums and communities can be a valuable space to connect with others living with CKD, share experiences, and ask questions.

Building a Network of Strength

By building a strong support network of loved ones and tapping into community resources, you create a safety net that can significantly improve your quality of life. This network can be a source of comfort, encouragement, and practical assistance, empowering you to navigate the challenges of CKD and live a fulfilling life.

CHAPTER FOUR

THE KIDNEY-FRIENDLY PLATE: NUTRITIONAL STRATEGIES FOR OPTIMAL HEALTH

4.1 DECODING FOOD LABELS: UNDERSTANDING PROTEIN, POTASSIUM, AND PHOSPHORUS

Navigating the supermarket can feel like a challenge when you have CKD, but don't worry! By understanding food labels, you can become a savvy shopper and make choices that support your kidney health. This chapter will help you focus on three key nutrients: protein, potassium, and phosphorus.

Mastering the Art of Label Reading

Food labels contain a wealth of information. Here's how to focus on the key sections relevant to your CKD diet:

Nutrition Facts Panel: This shows the calories, nutrients, and vitamins in a serving of food.

Serving Size: Pay close attention to this, as all nutrient amounts are listed per serving. It's easy to underestimate how much you're actually consuming!

Grams (g), Milligrams (mg), and Percent Daily Value (% DV): Nutrients are listed in grams for larger amounts and milligrams for smaller amounts. The % DV indicates how much a serving contributes to your daily needs.

Protein Power: But Moderation is Key

Protein is essential for building and repairing tissues, but too much can strain your kidneys. Here's what to keep in mind:

Understanding Protein Content: Look at the grams of protein per serving. Your doctor or dietitian will recommend how much protein you should consume based on your CKD stage.

Spreading Out Your Protein Intake: Distribute your protein consumption throughout the day rather than eating large amounts at once.

Choosing Protein Sources Wisely: opt for lean protein sources like fish, poultry (without skin), skinless chicken breast, beans, lentils, and low-fat dairy products. Limit red meat and processed meats, as they are often high in protein and phosphorus.

Potassium: A Balancing Act

Potassium is crucial for muscle function and nerve transmission, but with advanced CKD, you may need to manage your intake. Here's how:

Checking Potassium Levels: Your doctor will monitor your potassium through blood tests and may advise limiting high-potassium foods.

Understanding Potassium Content: Check the milligrams of potassium per serving.

Potassium Powerhouses: Fruits and vegetables are generally high in potassium. Common high-potassium foods include bananas, oranges, potatoes, tomatoes, and leafy greens.

Taming the Phosphorus Monster

Phosphorus is essential for bone health but can cause complications in CKD. Here's how to manage it:

Mind the Milligrams: Check the milligrams of phosphorus per serving. Your doctor or dietitian will recommend a phosphorus intake limit.

Phosphorus Powerhouses: Dairy products, processed meats, some nuts and seeds, and certain sodas are high in phosphorus. Look for alternatives or limit these foods.

Phosphorus Binding Medications: Your doctor may prescribe medications to help bind phosphorus in your digestive tract, preventing its absorption.

Beyond the Label: Tips for Savvy Shopping

Here are additional tips to make grocery shopping easier:

Plan Your Meals: Create a meal plan with kidney-friendly choices and check food labels beforehand.

Read Ingredient Lists: Look for hidden sources of protein, potassium, and phosphorus in processed foods.

Compare Brands: Nutrient amounts can vary between brands, even for the same type of food.

Ask for Help: Your dietitian can guide you in choosing appropriate foods and reading labels effectively.

Decoding food labels takes practice. With this knowledge and some planning, you can confidently navigate the grocery store, choosing foods that support your kidney health and overall well-being.

4.2 Creating a Delicious and Nutritious Diet for CKD

Living with CKD often means navigating dietary restrictions, but that doesn't mean your meals have to be bland or boring. This chapter will help you create delicious and nutritious dishes that support your kidney health while delighting your taste buds.

Embracing Flavor Without the Guilt

Spices and herbs are your best friends in the CKD kitchen. Dive into the vibrant world of spices like cumin, coriander, turmeric, and garlic powder. They add depth and complexity to your dishes without adding sodium or potassium. Fresh or dried herbs like basil, oregano, parsley, and thyme can also work wonders.

Beyond Salt: Exploring Flavor Enhancers

Sodium restriction is a cornerstone of a CKD diet, but you don't have to sacrifice flavor. Here are some alternatives to enhance your dishes:

- Lemon Juice and Zest: A squeeze of fresh lemon juice can brighten up your dishes and add a tangy kick.
- Vinegars: From balsamic to apple cider vinegar, explore different types to add acidity and depth of flavor.
- Black Pepper: Freshly ground black pepper adds heat and complexity without any sodium.
- Onion and Garlic: These versatile ingredients add a savory base to many dishes.
- Sugar Substitutes: If you have diabetes or need to manage blood sugar, use sugar substitutes approved by your doctor to add sweetness to your meals.

Protein Powerhouses: Making Smart Choices

Protein is essential, but for CKD, moderation and smart choices are key. Here are some delicious protein options:

- Fish: Fatty fish like salmon, tuna, and sardines are packed with omega-3 fatty acids, beneficial for heart health.

- Skinless Chicken and Turkey Breast: Lean protein sources that can be cooked in various ways.

- Eggs: A good source of protein and other essential nutrients. Enjoy them boiled, poached, or scrambled.

- Beans and Lentils: Plant-based protein powerhouses that are also high in fiber.

- Low-Fat Dairy Products: Options like Greek yogurt or low-fat milk provide protein and calcium.

- Potassium and Phosphorus: Making Informed Swaps

Some fruits and vegetables are high in potassium and phosphorus, but plenty of delicious options fit within your CKD diet. Here are some tips:

Potassium:

- Fruits: Berries, apples, grapes, and pears are generally lower in potassium compared to bananas, oranges, and cantaloupe.
- Vegetables: Green beans, asparagus, cabbage, and cauliflower are good choices.

Phosphorus:

Limit Dairy Products: Focus on low-fat options and consume them in moderation.

- Choose Lean Protein Sources: opt for fish and skinless chicken or turkey breast over red meat and processed meats.
- Enjoy Whole Grains: Brown rice, quinoa, and whole-wheat bread are good choices, but be mindful of portion sizes.

Embrace Cooking at Home: It's Rewarding!

Cooking at home allows you to control ingredients and portion sizes. Here are some tips to make it easier:

- Plan Your Meals: Helps you avoid unhealthy choices when you're short on time.
- Prepare in Advance: Chop vegetables, cook protein sources, or prepare whole grains ahead of time to save effort during the week.
- Batch Cooking: Make a large pot of soup or chili on the weekend for easy meals throughout the week.
- Explore Online Resources: Numerous websites and cookbooks are dedicated to creating delicious CKD-friendly meals.

A healthy CKD diet can be a delicious and sustainable journey. Experiment with flavors, explore new recipes, and don't be afraid to get creative in the kitchen. With a little planning and the right guidance, you can enjoy a satisfying and nutritious diet that supports your well-being.

4.3 Culinary Adventures: Adapting Favorite Recipes for Kidney Health

Missing your favorite comfort foods after a CKD diagnosis? Don't worry! With a bit of creativity and these handy tips, you can transform your favorite recipes into kidney-friendly masterpieces.

The Art of Recipe Adaptation: A Culinary Transformation

Think of adapting recipes as a culinary adventure. Here's how to approach it:

Deconstruct the Recipe: Break down your favorite recipe into its basic components – protein, vegetables, starches, and flavorings.

Identify Areas for Adjustment: Look for ingredients that might be high in protein, potassium, or phosphorus, depending on your specific needs.

Explore CKD-Friendly Alternatives: Find delicious substitutes for high-potassium or high-phosphorus ingredients. There are often multiple options to explore!

Spice Up Your Life: Don't forget the magic of spices and herbs. They can add depth and complexity to your dishes without adding sodium or potassium.

Protein Power: Making Smart Swaps

Protein is essential, but for CKD, moderation and choosing the right sources is key. Here are some swaps you can consider:

- Swap Red Meat for Fish: Fatty fish like salmon, tuna, and sardines are delicious and packed with omega-3 fatty acids.
- Replace High-Protein Meats with Beans and Lentils: These plant-based powerhouses are high in fiber and protein, making you feel fuller for longer.
- opt for Skinless, Lean Chicken or Turkey Breast: These are versatile protein sources that can be cooked in various ways.
- Explore Ground Turkey or Chicken: They can be used in place of beef in many recipes like burgers, tacos, or chili.

- Taming Potassium and Phosphorus: Finding Delicious Substitutes

Here are some tips for adapting recipes that might be high in potassium or phosphorus:

Potassium:

- Fruits: Swap bananas, oranges, or cantaloupe for berries, apples, grapes, or pears, which are generally lower in potassium.

- Vegetables: opt for green beans, asparagus, cabbage, or cauliflower instead of high-potassium vegetables like potatoes or tomatoes. You might need to adjust cooking times depending on the chosen substitutes.

Phosphorus:

- Limit Dairy Products: Focus on low-fat options and consume them in moderation. Consider using smaller amounts of cheese or yogurt in recipes.

- Choose Lean Protein Sources: opt for fish and skinless chicken or turkey breast over red meat and processed meats, which are often higher in phosphorus.

- Explore Whole Grains in Moderation: Brown rice, quinoa, and whole-wheat bread are good choices, but be mindful of portion sizes. You can sometimes use cauliflower rice as a low-carb alternative.

Sodium Savvy: Reducing Salt Without Sacrificing Flavor

Sodium restriction is often a cornerstone of a CKD diet. But that doesn't mean your food has to be bland! Here are some strategies:

- Rely on Herbs and Spices: Explore the vibrant world of spices like cumin, coriander, turmeric, and garlic powder. They add depth and complexity without adding sodium.

- Embrace Fresh Herbs: Fresh or dried herbs like basil, oregano, parsley, and thyme can work wonders, adding a fragrant touch to your dishes.

- Use Acidic Ingredients: A squeeze of fresh lemon juice can brighten up your dishes and add a tangy kick. Experiment with different vinegars like balsamic or apple cider vinegar for a touch of acidity.

- Explore Salt Substitutes: If approved by your doctor, consider using potassium chloride-based salt substitutes to add a salty flavor without adding extra sodium.

The Fun Part: Experimentation and Personalization

Remember, adapting recipes is a journey of discovery. Don't be afraid to experiment with different flavors and ingredients. Here are some additional tips:

Start with Small Changes: Modify one or two ingredients at a time and see how it affects the overall taste.

Taste as You Go: Adjust seasonings throughout the cooking process to ensure your dish is flavorful but not overly salty.

Embrace Online Resources: There are numerous websites and cookbooks dedicated to creating delicious CKD-friendly meals. Use them for inspiration and guidance.

Make it a Family Affair: Get your loved ones involved in the kitchen. Adapting recipes can be a fun and rewarding activity to do together.

Adapting your favorite recipes allows you to enjoy familiar flavors while staying on track with your CKD diet. Healthy eating doesn't have to be bland or restrictive. With a little creativity and these tips, you can embark on a culinary adventure, transforming your meals into delicious and kidney-friendly masterpieces!

CHAPTER FIVE

MOVE YOUR BODY, EMPOWER YOUR MIND: EXERCISE STRATEGIES FOR CKD

5.1 FINDING YOUR FIT: EXERCISE OPTIONS FOR DIFFERENT ABILITIES

Exercise might not be the first thing you think of when managing CKD, but it's a powerful tool that can boost your overall well-being, energy levels, and even help manage your condition. The best part? There's an exercise option for everyone, regardless of your physical abilities.

The Power of Movement: Why Exercise Matters for CKD

Here's how exercise benefits people with CKD:

Improved Blood Sugar Control: Exercise helps your body use insulin more effectively, which is especially beneficial if you have diabetes, a common condition alongside CKD.

Reduced Blood Pressure: Regular physical activity can help lower blood pressure, reducing the risk of heart disease and stroke.

Stronger Bones and Muscles: Exercise helps maintain muscle mass and bone density, which can be crucial for preventing fractures as CKD progresses.

Improved Mood and Energy Levels: Physical activity releases endorphins, which can boost your mood and combat fatigue.

Better Sleep: Regular exercise can improve sleep quality, leading to increased energy levels throughout the day.

Finding Your Exercise Groove: Activities for Every Body

The key to sticking with an exercise routine is finding activities you enjoy. Here are some options based on your abilities:

Low-Impact Activities:

Walking: Simple and accessible, walking can be done almost anywhere. Start slow and gradually increase the duration and intensity.

Swimming: Gentle on your joints and a great way to cool down on a hot day.

Yoga: Gentle stretching and breathing exercises improve flexibility, balance, and overall well-being.

Tai Chi: This mind-body practice combines slow, gentle movements with deep breathing, promoting relaxation and stress reduction.

Moderate-Intensity Activities:

Biking: Whether outdoors or on a stationary bike, cycling is great for cardiovascular health.

Dancing: Put on your favorite music and dance! It's a fun and social way to get some exercise.

Water Aerobics: A low-impact activity that's easy on your joints and a great way to cool down during your workout.

Strength Training:

Building muscle mass is essential for overall health. You can use bodyweight exercises like squats, lunges, and push-ups, or light weights or resistance bands.

Listen to Your Body: Essential Tips for Safety

Here are some key things to remember when starting an exercise routine:

Get Clearance from Your Doctor: Always consult your doctor before starting any new exercise program, especially if you have CKD. They can guide you on safe and appropriate activities.

Start Slow and Gradually Increase Intensity: Begin with low-intensity exercises for short durations and gradually increase as your fitness improves.

Listen to Your Body: Pay attention to your body's signals. If you experience any pain or discomfort, stop the activity and consult your doctor.

Hydration is Key: Drink plenty of water before, during, and after your workout to stay hydrated.

Find a Buddy: Exercising with a friend or family member can make it more fun and motivating.

Adapting Activities for Different Abilities

The beauty of exercise is its adaptability. Here are some ways to modify activities for different abilities:

Limited Mobility: If walking is difficult, consider using a walker or cane for support. You can also try chair exercises or gentle yoga poses.

Balance Issues: If balance is a concern, start with exercises that can be done while holding onto a wall or chair for support. Water aerobics is another great option for people with balance problems.

Pain Management: If you experience pain, talk to your doctor about modifications to your exercise routine. Low-impact activities like swimming or water aerobics might be a better choice.

Embrace the Journey: Exercise is a Lifelong Commitment

Exercise isn't just about achieving a specific goal; it's about incorporating movement into your daily life for long-term well-being. Here are some motivational tips:

Set Realistic Goals: Start small and celebrate your achievements, no matter how big or small.

Find Activities You Enjoy: Exercise shouldn't feel like a chore. Choose activities you look forward to doing.

Track Your Progress: Seeing your progress can be a great motivator. Keep a log of your workouts or use a fitness tracker.

By making exercise a regular part of your routine, you can improve your quality of life and better manage your CKD. Enjoy the journey and embrace the benefits of staying active!

5.2 Beyond the Gym: Building Activity into Your Daily Life

Finding time for dedicated exercise sessions is great, but the benefits of movement go beyond the gym. Here's the good news: incorporating small pockets of activity throughout your day can significantly enhance your overall well-being and support your CKD management.

Small Steps, Big Impact: Sneaking Activity into Your Day

Making physical activity a sustainable part of your life with CKD involves integrating it seamlessly into your daily routine. Here are some clever strategies:

Become a NEAT Ninja: NEAT stands for Non-Exercise Activity Thermogenesis, which refers to the calories you burn through everyday activities beyond structured exercise. Simple actions like taking the stairs instead of the elevator, parking further away, or pacing while on the phone all add up. Every little bit counts!

Tame the TV Monster: Use commercial breaks as an opportunity to move! Stretch, do some jumping jacks, or walk around the house during commercials to break up prolonged sitting.

The Active Commuter: If possible, incorporate walking, cycling, or scooting into your commute. It's a great way to add some activity into your morning and evening routine.

The Active Workstation: Sitting for long periods can be detrimental to your health. If possible, invest in a standing desk, or take frequent short walking breaks throughout your workday. Under-desk ellipticals can also help you move your legs while you work.

The Household Hustle: Turn daily chores into mini-workouts. Wash your car by hand, dance while cleaning, or park further away at the grocery store and carry your groceries – all these actions contribute to your daily activity level.

Making Activity a Social Affair: Move with Your Loved Ones

Exercising with friends or family can keep you motivated and make physical activity more enjoyable. Here are some ideas:

Buddy Up for Walks: Find a friend or family member to walk with regularly. It's a fantastic way to catch up, enjoy nature, and get some exercise together.

Join a Group Fitness Class: Look for low-impact group fitness classes like yoga, tai chi, or water aerobics. It's a social way to stay active and meet new people with similar interests.

Active Family Fun: Plan weekend activities that involve movement, like hiking, biking, or playing games in the park. Make it a fun family outing that everyone can enjoy.

Technology as Your Fitness Partner

Numerous apps and wearable fitness trackers can help you monitor your activity levels and stay motivated. Here's how technology can be your ally:

Fitness Trackers: Wearable devices track your steps, distance walked, and calories burned. They can motivate you to reach your daily activity goals.

Exercise Apps: Many apps offer guided workouts, yoga routines, or mindfulness exercises that you can do at home with minimal equipment.

Online Fitness Communities: Join online communities dedicated to fitness or CKD management. These can provide inspiration, motivation, and a platform to connect with others on a similar journey.

To reap the benefits of physical activity, consistency is crucial. Even small bursts of activity throughout your day can accumulate and make a significant difference in your overall well-being. Don't get discouraged if you miss a day or two – just get back on track the next day!

5.3 The Mind-Body Connection: Exercise for Stress Management and Well-being

Living with CKD can bring about its fair share of stress. From managing your diet to keeping track of medications and monitoring the progression of the disease, it's understandable to feel overwhelmed. However, here's a silver lining: exercise isn't just about physical health; it's a potent tool for managing stress and nurturing emotional well-being. In this chapter, we delve into the mind-body connection and explore how integrating physical activity into your routine can help you tackle stress and cultivate a positive mindset.

The Stress-CKD Connection: A Vicious Cycle

Chronic stress can wreak havoc on both your physical and mental well-being. When stress takes hold, your body releases hormones like cortisol, which can:

- Increase blood pressure
- Elevate blood sugar levels
- Weaken the immune system

These factors can further complicate CKD management, creating a vicious cycle where stress exacerbates CKD, and CKD, in turn, becomes a source of stress.

Exercise: Your Stress-Busting Ally

The bright side is that exercise can serve as a potent antidote to stress. Here's how physical activity can lend a helping hand:

Boosts Mood and Reduces Anxiety: Exercise triggers the release of endorphins, which are hormones known for their mood-enhancing effects. Regular physical activity can help alleviate feelings of anxiety and foster a sense of well-being.

Improves Sleep Quality: Stress often disrupts sleep, but exercise can promote quicker and more restful sleep. Quality sleep is vital for managing stress and overall health.

Increases Focus and Clarity: Physical activity enhances cognitive function, helping you feel more alert and focused. This can be particularly beneficial for handling the challenges of living with CKD.

Provides a Healthy Outlet: Exercise offers a constructive way to channel negative emotions like frustration or anger.

It allows you to redirect your focus onto your body and release pent-up tension.

Finding Your Exercise Oasis: Activities for Stress Relief

Harnessing exercise for stress management begins with finding activities that resonate with you. Here are some options to explore:

Mind-Body Practices: Yoga, tai chi, and meditation blend physical movement with mindfulness techniques, fostering relaxation and stress reduction.

Activities in Nature: Spending time outdoors, whether walking in the park, gardening, or hiking, can offer a soothing escape and a chance to reconnect with nature.

Social Activities: Engage in group fitness classes, dance sessions with friends, or play a sport you enjoy. Combining social interaction with physical activity can be a potent stress reliever.

Building a Sustainable Exercise Routine for Stress Management

Here are some pointers for incorporating exercise into your routine to manage stress effectively:

Start Small and Gradually Increase: Avoid the temptation to dive in too deep from the get-go. Begin with short bursts of activity and slowly ramp up the duration and intensity.

Choose Enjoyable Activities: Exercise shouldn't feel like a chore. opt for activities that you genuinely look forward to, whether it's grooving to your favorite tunes or strolling through picturesque scenery.

Schedule Your Workouts: Treat your exercise regimen as you would any other vital commitment. Block out time in your calendar and strive to stick to it consistently.

Find an Exercise Buddy: Having a workout partner can provide motivation and make physical activity more enjoyable.

Listen to Your Body: Pay heed to your body's cues. If you feel overwhelmed or stressed during a workout, take a breather or modify the activity.

To reap the stress-relieving benefits of exercise, consistency is paramount. Even brief bouts of activity on most days of the week can wield a significant impact on your emotional well-being. If you miss a day or two, don't be disheartened – simply pick up where you left off the next day!

CHAPTER SIX

SLEEP, STRESS, AND YOUR KIDNEYS: CULTIVATING A HEALTHY LIFESTYLE

6.1 THE POWER OF REST: PRIORITIZING QUALITY SLEEP FOR CKD

Ever find yourself struggling to get a good night's sleep, especially since your CKD diagnosis? You're definitely not alone. Sleep issues are a common challenge for folks dealing with CKD. But here's the silver lining: focusing on quality sleep isn't just about feeling refreshed—it's a vital part of managing CKD and staying healthy overall.

Why Sleep Matters for CKD

Sleep is crucial for both our physical and mental health. While we catch some Z's, our bodies get to work repairing tissues, regulating hormones, and even sorting through memories. For those with CKD, getting enough shut-eye is extra important for a few key reasons:

Blood Pressure Control: Solid sleep helps keep blood pressure in check, a big deal for CKD warriors. Skimping on sleep can lead to blood pressure fluctuations, putting more stress on your kidneys.

Blood Sugar Management: Sleep deprivation can mess with the hormones that control blood sugar levels. This can be especially tough if you're managing diabetes alongside CKD.

Immune System Support: Chronic sleep issues can weaken your immune system, leaving you more vulnerable to getting sick. And for folks with CKD, who already have weakened immunity, this is a big concern.

Boosted Energy Levels: Fatigue is a common CKD symptom. But catching quality Z's can help you feel more energized during the day, making it easier to tackle your daily tasks and treatment routines.

Understanding Sleep Problems in CKD

A bunch of things can throw a wrench in your sleep plans when you've got CKD:

Restless Legs Syndrome (RLS): This condition makes you feel the urge to move your legs, often worse at night, which can make falling and staying asleep tough.

Frequent Urination (Nocturia): Needing to pee multiple times a night can really mess with your sleep. This can happen due to things like drinking too much before bed, certain meds, or uncontrolled blood sugar.

Sleep Apnea: Folks with CKD are at a higher risk for this disorder, which causes breathing pauses during sleep and can leave you feeling groggy during the day.

Pain and Discomfort: Nerve pain or itchy skin can make it hard to drift off or get comfy at night.

Stress and Anxiety: Dealing with CKD can be super stressful, and that stress can make it tough to catch quality Z's.

Creating a Sleep Sanctuary: Tips for Better Sleep

Here are some tricks to help you improve your sleep habits and get some quality shut-eye:

Stick to a Sleep Schedule: Aim to hit the hay and wake up at the same time every day to help regulate your body's internal clock.

Wind Down: Establish a relaxing bedtime routine with activities like a warm bath, reading, or listening to soothing tunes. Ditch the screens at least an hour before bedtime to avoid messing with your sleep patterns.

Set the Scene: Make your bedroom a cozy haven by keeping it dark, quiet, and cool. Invest in blackout curtains, earplugs, and a comfy mattress and pillows.

Watch Your Intake: Cut back on caffeine in the afternoon and evening, as it can interfere with sleep. While a nightcap might seem relaxing, booze can mess with your sleep quality in the long run.

Get Moving: Regular exercise can help you sleep better. Just avoid intense workouts too close to bedtime, as they can rev you up instead of winding you down.

Chill Out: Stress can wreck your sleep, so try relaxation techniques like deep breathing or meditation before bed to help calm your mind and body.

Talk to Your Doc: If sleep troubles persist, chat with your doctor. They can help sass out any underlying issues and suggest treatments or therapies to improve your sleep quality.

Working with Your Doctor to Improve Sleep

If you're still tossing and turning despite your best efforts, it's crucial to loop in your doc. They can help pinpoint any underlying conditions contributing to your sleep woes and recommend treatments or meds to help you catch those Z's.

Remember: Quality Sleep is a Game-Changer for Your Health

Getting good sleep isn't just a nice-to-have—it's a must when you're dealing with CKD. By making some tweaks to your routine and tackling any underlying issues, you can boost your sleep quality and reap the rewards when it comes to managing your CKD and living your best life.

6.2 Taming the Tiger: Effective Stress Management Techniques

Dealing with stress is a universal experience, and for those with CKD, it can feel like an unwelcome companion that just won't leave. But fear not! Just like we can train a wild tiger, there are effective ways to manage stress and find inner peace. This chapter is all about arming you with tools to tackle stress head-on and boost your overall well-being.

Understanding Stress: The Body's Response

When faced with stress, your body kicks into fight-or-flight mode, releasing hormones like adrenaline and cortisol to prepare you for action. But in today's world, stress is often chronic, and this constant activation of the fight-or-flight response can take a toll on your physical and mental health, especially for those with CKD.

The Impact of Chronic Stress on CKD

For CKD patients, chronic stress can worsen existing health issues:

Blood Pressure Spikes: Stress can temporarily raise blood pressure, putting extra strain on already stressed kidneys.

Weakened Immunity: Chronic stress can suppress the immune system, leaving you more vulnerable to infections—a big concern for CKD patients.

Blood Sugar Swings: Stress hormones can disrupt insulin use, leading to higher blood sugar levels, particularly problematic for those with diabetes.

Sleep Troubles: Stress can mess with your sleep, making it hard to get quality rest—a vital part of managing CKD.

Taking Control: Stress Management Techniques

The good news? You're not powerless against stress. Here are some techniques to add to your stress-fighting toolkit:

Relaxation Techniques: Deep breathing, progressive muscle relaxation, and meditation can activate your body's relaxation response.

Mindfulness Practices: Paying attention to the present moment without judgment can help you disconnect from stress.

Cognitive Behavioral Therapy (CBT): This therapy helps you challenge negative thought patterns contributing to stress.

Journaling: Writing down your thoughts can be a helpful way to process stress.

Connecting with Loved Ones: Spending time with supportive friends and family can provide comfort and reduce stress.

Laughter: Engage in activities that make you laugh—it's a powerful stress reliever.

Engaging in Enjoyable Activities: Make time for hobbies and activities you love.

Finding What Works for You

The key is finding what stress-busting strategies work best for you. Experiment with different techniques and stick with what resonates most. Whether it's deep breathing, meditation, or a good laugh, find what helps you tame the stress tiger.

Making Stress Management a Priority

Remember, managing stress isn't just a nice-to-have—it's essential, especially for those with CKD. By incorporating these techniques into your daily life, you can take control of stress, boost your well-being, and effectively manage your CKD journey.

6.3 Building Resilience: Developing a Positive Mindset for Living Well with CKD

Living with a chronic condition like CKD comes with its share of hurdles. Feeling fear, frustration, or even anger is completely normal. But here's the silver lining: embracing a positive mindset, also known as resilience, can be a game-changer. It empowers you to tackle challenges head-on, adapt to changes, and find fulfillment despite CKD.

Understanding Resilience and its Impact

Resilience is all about bouncing back from tough times, dealing with stress, and keeping a hopeful outlook. It's not about pretending everything's perfect but about-facing difficulties with optimism. Here's why it's crucial for living well with CKD:

Enhanced Quality of Life: A positive mindset can brighten your outlook, helping you focus on the good stuff and savor life's moments.

Improved Treatment Adherence: Staying committed to your treatment plan is key for managing CKD effectively. Resilience keeps you motivated and determined, even when the going gets tough.

Lowered Stress and Anxiety: Dealing with a chronic illness can be overwhelming, but resilience helps you handle stress and anxiety better, promoting overall well-being.

Better Social Connections: Feeling positive boosts your confidence and social interactions. It helps you connect with others and build a support system you can rely on.

Building Your Resilience Toolbox: Tips for a Positive Mindset

Here are some practical strategies to cultivate resilience:

Gratitude Practice: Take a moment each day to count your blessings. It shifts your focus away from negativity.

Positive Self-Talk: Swap out self-doubt with encouraging words. Instead of "I can't," try "I can find a way through this."

Focus on Control: Concentrate on what you can influence, like lifestyle choices and stress management.

Embrace Growth: See setbacks as opportunities for growth and learning.

Celebrate Wins: Even small victories deserve recognition—they keep you moving forward.

Find Meaning: Connect with what matters to you, whether it's hobbies, volunteering, or pursuing passions.

Seek Support: Lean on friends, family, and healthcare pros when you need a hand.

Resilience is a journey, not a Destination

Building resilience takes time. Some days will be easier than others, and that's okay. Keep practicing these strategies, and you'll gradually develop a sunnier outlook and a knack for tackling challenges like a pro.

.

CHAPTER SEVEN

Medication Management: Understanding and Adhering to Your Treatment Plan

7.1 DEMYSTIFYING MEDICATIONS: COMMON DRUGS USED IN CKD TREATMENT

Medications play a crucial role in managing CKD, helping control various aspects of the disease like blood pressure, blood sugar levels, and anemia. While the idea of medication might feel overwhelming, knowing their purpose and how they work puts you in the driver's seat of your CKD treatment.

Partnering with Your Doctor: A Team Effort

You're not alone in this journey. Your doctor is your ally in CKD management, working with you to tailor a treatment plan that suits your needs. Here's what you can expect:

Open Communication: Don't hesitate to discuss any questions or concerns about your medications with your doctor. Talk about potential side effects and how the meds fit into your daily life.

Understanding Your Meds: Ask your doctor to break down how each medication functions and its role in your overall treatment strategy. Knowledge is empowering!

Medication Adherence: Taking your meds exactly as prescribed is vital for effective CKD management. Work with your doctor to stay on track, especially if you're juggling multiple prescriptions.

Common Medications in CKD Treatment:

Let's break down some typical medications used:

Blood Pressure Meds: ACE inhibitors, ARBs, diuretics, and calcium channel blockers can help keep your blood pressure in check.

Blood Sugar Control: For diabetes, you might need meds like metformin, DPP-4 inhibitors, or SGLT2 inhibitors to manage blood sugar levels.

Anemia Management: ESAs and iron supplements can boost red blood cell production to combat anemia.

Phosphate Binders: These meds help regulate phosphorus levels in your blood as CKD progresses.

Vitamin D Supplements: To address vitamin D deficiencies common in CKD, your doctor might recommend supplements for bone health.

Key Points to Remember:

This list isn't exhaustive; your doctor will tailor medications to your unique situation and CKD stage.

- Be mindful of potential side effects for each medication and discuss any concerns with your doctor.
- Never tweak your medication regimen without consulting your doctor first.

Taking Charge of Your Health:

Understanding your CKD meds puts you in control. By teaming up with your doctor, asking questions, and sticking to your prescribed regimen, you're equipped to manage CKD effectively and lead a fulfilling life.

7.2 Working with Your Doctor: Optimizing Your Medication Regimen

Medications are pivotal in managing CKD, keeping various disease aspects in check and averting complications. However, managing a medication routine can be daunting. This section is all about empowering you to actively engage in your CKD treatment by fostering a collaborative bond with your doctor to fine-tune your medication plan.

Cultivating a Strong Doctor-Patient Relationship: Communication is Key

The cornerstone of an effective medication plan rests on transparent and candid communication with your doctor. Here's how to build a robust doctor-patient rapport that serves your CKD management well:

Speak Up and Ask Away: Don't hold back from expressing any worries or queries about medications. Whether it's about potential side effects, how meds might affect your daily life, or confusion about their purpose, airing your concerns is crucial.

Knowledge is Power: Request your doctor to break down how each medication operates and its specific role in your treatment blueprint. Grasping the ins and outs of your meds empowers you to be a well-informed and proactive participant in your healthcare.

Honesty Wins Every Time: Be transparent with your doctor about your medication adherence. Share any hurdles you encounter in sticking to the prescribed regimen, and collaborate on finding solutions together.

Optimizing Your Medication Plan: A Team Effort

Consider these vital aspects when collaborating with your doctor to fine-tune your medication regimen:

Tailored Treatment: CKD treatment isn't one-size-fits-all. Your doctor will factor in your unique requirements, CKD stage, and any coexisting health conditions when determining the most suitable medications and dosages.

Regular Evaluations and Tweaks: With CKD progression or changes in your health status, your medication regimen might need tweaking. Regular check-ins with your doctor are vital to address concerns and ensure your meds are still on point.

Managing Side Effects: Many meds come with potential side effects. Be aware of these and discuss them openly with your doctor. Don't suffer in silence – your doctor can help mitigate side effects or explore alternative meds if needed.

Strategies for Effective Medication Management:

Here are some practical pointers to help you stay on top of your medication regimen:

Establish a Routine: Take your meds at consistent times each day, be it with meals, at bedtime, or in the morning. This consistency helps ward off missed doses.

Set Reminders: Use alarms on your phone or a pill organizer with daily compartments. Visual cues can be invaluable in staying on course.

Maintain a Med List: Keep an updated inventory of all your meds, including names, dosages, and schedules. This comes in handy when communicating with different healthcare providers.

Travel Prep: When traveling, plan ahead. Ensure you pack enough meds for your trip and carry them in your carry-on bag to dodge baggage delays. Discuss any potential medication tweaks due to time zone shifts with your doctor.

Involve Your Support Circle: Share your medication plan with a trusted loved one. They can serve as a gentle reminder system and offer support if you encounter any hurdles.

Your doctor is your ally in CKD management. By fostering open communication and collaboration, you can fine-tune your medication regimen, arm yourself with knowledge, and seize control of your health journey.

7.3 Overcoming Challenges: Strategies for Adherence and Avoiding Side Effects

Taking medications as prescribed is crucial for effectively managing CKD. However, sticking to a medication regimen can be challenging. This chapter equips you with strategies to overcome common hurdles and navigate potential side effects, empowering you to stay on track with your treatment plan.

Understanding Medication Adherence and Why it Matters

Medication adherence refers to taking your medications exactly as prescribed by your doctor, including the correct dosage and frequency. Here's why adherence is so important for CKD management:

Optimizes Treatment Benefits: Following your medication regimen allows them to work effectively, controlling blood pressure, blood sugar levels, and other aspects of CKD.

Reduces Risk of Complications: Consistent medication use can help prevent complications associated with CKD, such as heart disease, stroke, and kidney failure.

Improves Quality of Life: By effectively managing your CKD, you can experience a better overall quality of life, with fewer symptoms and increased energy levels.

Common Challenges to Medication Adherence

Several factors can make it difficult to stick to your medication regimen. Here are some common challenges and solutions:

Complexity of Regimen: Taking multiple medications at different times throughout the day can be confusing.

Solution: Develop a routine and use reminders like alarms or a pill organizer to stay on track.

Side Effects: Some medications can cause unpleasant side effects, tempting you to skip doses.

Solution: Discuss side effects with your doctor. They might be able to adjust the dosage, prescribe a different medication, or offer strategies for managing side effects.

Cost Concerns: The cost of medications can be a significant burden.

Solution: Talk to your doctor about generic alternatives or explore patient assistance programs that can help with medication costs.

Forgetfulness: Life gets busy, and sometimes you might forget to take your medications.

Solution: Set reminders, link medication intake to daily activities (e.g., take medication with breakfast), or involve a trusted family member or friend as a gentle reminder system.

Lack of Understanding: If you don't understand the purpose of your medications, you might be less motivated to take them consistently.

Solution: Ask your doctor to explain how each medication works and its role in your overall CKD management.

Effective Communication is Key

Open communication with your doctor is vital for overcoming challenges and maintaining medication adherence. Here are some tips:

Be Honest: Discuss any difficulties you face with taking medications as prescribed. Don't be embarrassed to share concerns about side effects, cost, or forgetfulness.

Ask Questions: Don't hesitate to ask your doctor about anything you don't understand regarding your medications. The more informed you are, the more empowered you feel to manage your CKD effectively.

Work Together: View your doctor as a partner in your CKD journey. Collaborate with them to find solutions for overcoming medication adherence challenges.

Proactive Strategies for Side Effect Management

While some side effects are unavoidable, there are ways to manage them and improve your medication adherence:

Discuss Side Effects with Your Doctor: Talk to your doctor about potential side effects and explore ways to minimize them. They might suggest taking medications with food, adjusting the timing of your dosage, or prescribing alternative medications with fewer side effects.

Lifestyle Modifications: Certain lifestyle changes can help manage side effects. For example, increasing water intake can help reduce constipation caused by some medications. Exercise can improve fatigue associated with other medications.

Over-the-Counter Relief: For some side effects, like nausea or headaches, over-the-counter medications can provide relief. However, always consult your doctor before taking any new medications, even over-the-counter ones, to avoid potential interactions.

Remember: Medication adherence is an ongoing process. There will be times when you face challenges. However, by understanding the importance of adherence, developing strategies to overcome hurdles, and proactively managing side effects, you can stay on track with your treatment plan and empower yourself to live well with CKD.

CHAPTER EIGHT

NAVIGATING TREATMENT OPTIONS: DIALYSIS AND BEYOND

8.1 UNDERSTANDING DIALYSIS: AN OVERVIEW OF TREATMENT OPTIONS

Kidney failure, the most advanced stage of CKD, occurs when your kidneys can no longer effectively filter waste products and excess fluid from your blood. Dialysis steps in as a lifesaving treatment, taking over this vital function and enabling you to maintain a vibrant and active lifestyle. This section delves into the various types of dialysis, equipping you with the knowledge to navigate this critical aspect of CKD management.

Why Dialysis is Essential

Healthy kidneys undertake several crucial functions, including:

Filtering Waste Products: Removing waste products like creatinine and urea from your blood.

Balancing Electrolytes: Maintaining the proper balance of electrolytes, crucial minerals for nerve and muscle function.

Regulating Blood Pressure: Controlling fluid levels in your body to regulate blood pressure.

Producing Red Blood Cells: Generating erythropoietin (EPO), a hormone vital for red blood cell production.

When kidneys fail, these functions falter. Waste products accumulate, electrolyte imbalances arise, blood pressure spikes, and anemia sets in. Dialysis steps in to replicate these essential kidney functions, ensuring your blood remains clean and balanced.

Types of Dialysis: Tailoring Treatment to You

Two main types of dialysis exist: hemodialysis and peritoneal dialysis. The choice between them hinges on factors like your overall health, lifestyle preferences, and vascular access.

HEMODIALYSIS:

Blood Removal: Your blood is drawn out via a needle or catheter placed in a surgically created access point, often in your arm.

Artificial Kidney (Dialyzer): Blood flows through a machine called a dialyzer, functioning as an artificial kidney to filter waste and excess fluid.

Cleansed Blood Return: After purification, the clean blood returns to your body through another needle or catheter.

Hemodialysis is typically done in a center thrice weekly for hours each session, though home options exist for more flexibility.

PERITONEAL DIALYSIS:

Dialysis Solution Insertion: Sterile fluid, known as dialysis solution, is introduced into your abdominal cavity through a catheter placed in your belly.

Waste Diffusion: Waste and fluid seep from your blood into the dialysis solution.

Solution Replacement: The used solution is drained, and fresh solution is instilled, typically multiple times daily or overnight while you sleep.

Peritoneal dialysis offers various schedules to align with your lifestyle.

Considering Your Options: Collaborating with Your Doctor

The decision on dialysis type involves mutual deliberation between you and your doctor. Factors like your health status, lifestyle, and vascular access are weighed to determine the most suitable choice. Your doctor will also consider your support system and home situation for peritoneal dialysis.

Preparing for Dialysis: Education and Support

Comprehensive training and support are indispensable, whether you opt for home dialysis or center-based sessions. Your healthcare team offers guidance on dialysis procedures, and support groups provide a platform to connect with others facing similar challenges.

Dialysis is a lifesaver, enabling you to lead a fulfilling life despite CKD. By comprehending the available options and collaborating with your doctor, you can select the treatment that aligns best with your needs and preferences.

8.2 Kidney Transplantation: A Gift of Life

For those grappling with advanced CKD, kidney transplantation emerges as a beacon of hope, promising a new lease on life and a substantial boost in overall well-being. In this section, we embark on an exploration of the realm of kidney transplantation, unraveling its intricacies, from comprehending the process and eligibility criteria to navigating the waitlist and preparing for the surgical procedure.

A Fresh Start: The Impact of Kidney Transplantation

Kidney transplantation entails the surgical transfer of a healthy kidney from a donor into your body. This transplanted kidney assumes the critical functions that your failing kidneys can no longer fulfill, such as filtering waste products, maintaining electrolyte balance, and regulating blood pressure.

Compared to dialysis, kidney transplantation offers several notable advantages:

Enhanced Quality of Life: Transplant recipients often report heightened energy levels, increased dietary flexibility, and a more adaptable lifestyle in contrast to dialysis.

Reduced Long-Term Complications: A functioning kidney aids in regulating blood pressure and hormone levels, potentially mitigating the risk of long-term complications linked to CKD, such as heart disease and bone issues.

Heightened Independence: Dialysis, particularly hemodialysis, necessitates frequent visits to a dialysis center. Conversely, kidney transplantation affords greater autonomy and control over your daily schedule.

The Gift of Life: Exploring Donor Options

Two primary avenues exist for kidney donation:

1. Living Donor: A living donor, whether a close acquaintance, family member, or altruistic stranger, voluntarily contributes one of their healthy kidneys.

Living donor transplants offer perks like the ability to pre-schedule surgery when a compatible kidney is available.

2. Deceased Donor: Deceased donor kidneys originate from individuals who have passed away but possess organs deemed suitable for transplantation. The wait time for a deceased donor kidney varies considerably based on factors such as blood type and geographical location.

The Transplant Evaluation Process: Are You a Candidate?

Eligibility for a kidney transplant hinges on a thorough evaluation by your healthcare provider. This evaluation encompasses:

Medical History Review: An assessment of your overall health and existing medical conditions to ascertain your suitability for surgery and post-transplant medication regimen.

Blood Tests: Crucial for determining blood type compatibility and identifying any underlying conditions that could affect transplant success.

Imaging Tests: Utilized to evaluate the condition of your remaining kidneys and blood vessels.

Psychological Evaluation: Essential for gauging your emotional readiness to undergo the transplant procedure and adhere to post-transplant care requirements.

The Waitlist Journey: Preparing for Your Transplant

Upon determination of eligibility, you're likely to be enlisted on a waitlist for a deceased donor kidney. Wait times vary, contingent upon factors like blood type and geographical location. During this waiting period, it's imperative to:

Maintain a Healthy Lifestyle: Adherence to a nutritious diet, regular exercise, and management of existing health conditions bolsters your overall health and fortifies your candidacy for transplantation.

Stay Informed: Equip yourself with knowledge about kidney transplantation, its associated risks and benefits, and the recovery process. Engage with your healthcare provider and partake in transplant education initiatives provided by your transplant center.

Build Your Support System: Forge a robust network comprising friends, family, and healthcare professionals who can offer emotional support, practical assistance during recuperation, and encouragement throughout the journey.

The Gift of Life: The Transplant Surgery and Beyond

Kidney transplant surgery, typically conducted under general anesthesia, is a significant procedure. The surgeon meticulously implants the donor kidney into your lower abdomen, establishing connections to your blood vessels and urinary system. Recovery spans several weeks, accompanied by lifelong adherence to immunosuppressive medications to stave off rejection of the transplanted kidney.

Living with a Transplanted Kidney: Embracing a Fresh Chapter

The journey post-transplant necessitates ongoing follow-up care with your transplant team. This entails regular check-ups, monitoring medication levels, and vigilant surveillance for any signs of rejection. Nevertheless, for many individuals, a successful kidney transplant heralds a revitalized sense of freedom, heightened vitality, and the capacity to relish life to its fullest.

Kidney transplantation presents a transformative opportunity. By grasping the intricacies of the process, eligibility criteria, and the journey ahead, you can approach this prospective treatment avenue armed with hope and empowerment. In the subsequent chapter, we delve into the pivotal role of nutrition in CKD management, delving into dietary adjustments, crafting balanced meal plans, and strategies for upholding optimal nutrition throughout your CKD voyage.

8.3 Making Informed Decisions: Exploring Your Treatment Choices

Chronic kidney disease (CKD) progresses over time, and as it does, treatment options may change. This section is all about helping you make informed decisions regarding dialysis and kidney transplantation, taking into account your unique circumstances, preferences, and overall health.

Grasping Your Choices: Dialysis vs. Transplantation

As kidney function declines, dialysis or transplantation emerge as the primary treatments to compensate for the essential functions your kidneys can no longer fulfill. Let's break down the key aspects of each:

DIALYSIS:

Lifesaving Treatment: Dialysis effectively removes waste products and excess fluid from your bloodstream, allowing you to maintain a fulfilling life.

Two Main Types: Hemodialysis involves blood filtration through a machine, either in a center or at home, while peritoneal dialysis utilizes your abdominal lining as a natural filter.

Considerations: Dialysis entails a significant time commitment, dietary adjustments, and ongoing monitoring. It's essential to discuss how these factors may impact your lifestyle with your healthcare provider.

KIDNEY TRANSPLANTATION:

The Gift of Life: A kidney transplant provides an opportunity for enhanced freedom and well-being as a healthy donor kidney assumes the functions of your failing kidneys.

Improved Quality of Life: Transplant recipients often report increased energy levels, greater dietary flexibility, and a more adaptable lifestyle compared to dialysis.

Eligibility and Waitlist: Not everyone is eligible for a transplant. A thorough evaluation is necessary, and wait times for deceased donor kidneys can vary widely.

Factors to Ponder When Making Your Decision

There's no one-size-fits-all solution when it comes to choosing between dialysis and transplantation. Your optimal choice will hinge on several factors, including:

Your Overall Health: Your healthcare provider will evaluate your overall health and any coexisting medical conditions to determine the suitability of dialysis or transplant surgery.

Lifestyle Preferences: Consider the time commitments and flexibility associated with each treatment option. While hemodialysis requires frequent center visits, peritoneal dialysis offers more flexibility but might influence your daily activities.

Support System: A robust support network is indispensable for both dialysis and transplantation. Assess the assistance available to you at home, particularly if you opt for peritoneal dialysis.

Your Values and Preferences: Engage in candid discussions with your doctor and loved ones regarding the potential advantages and drawbacks of each option. Ultimately, your decision should align with your values and desired quality of life.

Transparent Communication: The Key to Enlightened Choices

Maintaining open and honest communication with your healthcare provider is paramount throughout your CKD journey. Here are some pointers for facilitating informed decision-making:

Ask Questions: Don't hesitate to seek clarification from your doctor about any aspect of dialysis, transplantation, or your specific circumstances that you find unclear.

Explore All Avenues: Delve into both dialysis and transplantation thoroughly, even if you initially lean towards one option. Understanding all possibilities empowers you to make the most informed decision.

Gather Additional Information: Reputable organizations like the National Kidney Foundation offer valuable educational resources on dialysis and transplantation. **Make the most of these resources to deepen your understanding**.

Consider a Second Opinion: If you harbor doubts or reservations, seeking a second opinion from another nephrologist (kidney specialist) can provide additional insights and bolster your confidence in your decision.

You're not alone in this journey. Your healthcare team is there to support and guide you through the decision-making process. By carefully weighing your options, asking pertinent questions, and expressing your concerns, you can make a well-informed decision that aligns with your individual needs and preferences for managing your CKD.

CHAPTER NINE

BUILDING A SUPPORT SYSTEM: SHARING YOUR JOURNEY WITH OTHERS

9.1 COMMUNICATION IS KEY: TALKING TO FAMILY AND FRIENDS ABOUT CKD

Living with chronic kidney disease (CKD) isn't just a personal journey—it affects your loved ones too. That's why open communication with family and friends is crucial for building a solid support system and navigating the emotional and practical aspects of life with CKD. This section provides you with strategies to start conversations about your condition, address their concerns, and foster understanding and support.

The Importance of Sharing: Why Communication Counts

Having conversations about CKD with your loved ones offers several benefits:

Reduced Stress and Burden: Keeping your feelings bottled up can be isolating and stressful. Sharing your diagnosis allows you to express yourself, easing some of the burden.

Building a Support System: Opening up lets your family and friends provide emotional support and practical assistance, helping you manage CKD more effectively.

Increased Understanding: Open communication helps your loved one's grasp CKD's impact on your life and how they can best support you.

Starting the Conversation: Tips for Breaking the Ice

Initiating a discussion about CKD might feel daunting. Here are some tips to help you get started:

Choose the Right Time and Place: Find a quiet, private setting where you can have an uninterrupted conversation.

Share Your Diagnosis: Be upfront about your diagnosis and the stage of your CKD.

Explain the Impact: Discuss how CKD affects your daily life, any limitations you face, and the treatment options you're considering.

Express Your Needs: Let them know what kind of support you require, whether it's emotional encouragement, assistance with tasks, or help with meal prep.

Addressing Concerns: Building Understanding

Your loved ones may have questions and worries about your CKD. Here's how you can address them:

Be Patient: Understand that they might not grasp everything about CKD right away. Answer their questions patiently and provide clear explanations.

Offer Reliable Resources: Point them towards reputable websites or patient support groups to deepen their understanding.

Clarify Misunderstandings: Correct any misconceptions they might have about CKD gently and provide accurate information.

Stay Positive: While CKD poses challenges, share your hope for the future and the positive steps you're taking to manage your condition.

Creating a Supportive Environment: Teamwork Matters

By involving your loved ones in your CKD journey, you create a supportive network:

Encourage Openness: Let them know they can approach you with any questions or concerns.

Delegate Tasks: Don't hesitate to ask for help with tasks like transportation or medication management.

Celebrate Together: Acknowledge your victories, big or small, with your support system. This reinforces a positive outlook and strengthens your bond.

Communication is a two-way street. By openly discussing your CKD with your loved ones, you build understanding, strengthen your support system, and empower them to be active participants in your wellness journey. In the next chapter, we'll delve into the importance of emotional well-being when living with CKD, exploring strategies for managing stress, coping with anxiety, and finding healthy ways to adjust to life with a chronic condition.

9.2 Finding Your Tribe: Connecting with Support Groups and Online Communities

Living with a chronic illness like CKD can often feel like you're navigating it alone. Questions, anxieties, and frustrations might swirl around, and it's tough when others can't fully grasp what you're going through. But fear not, as this section sheds light on the importance of plugging into support groups and online communities, where you'll find a sense of camaraderie and a wealth of resources for your CKD journey.

Why Support Groups Matter

Support groups offer a special haven where you can connect with others who truly get the ins and outs of living with CKD. Here's why they're so invaluable:

Shared Experiences: Bonding with fellow CKD warriors lets you openly discuss your experiences, feelings, and worries in a safe, understanding space.

Combat Isolation: It's easy to feel alone in this journey, but support groups help combat isolation by providing a sense of community and belonging.

Learning Opportunities: You'll glean invaluable insights and tips from those who've been navigating CKD for longer periods.

Emotional Lifeline: These groups offer a platform to express your emotions freely and receive encouragement and understanding from folks facing similar challenges.

Finding Your Tribe: Navigating Support Group Options

Finding the right support group isn't a one-size-fits-all affair. Here's how to hunt down a group that suits your needs:

Doctor's Orders: Your healthcare provider might be aware of local support groups tailored for CKD patients.

National Kidney Foundation: Use the NKF's patient services locator tool to scout support groups in your area or online.

Kidney Organizations: Organizations like AAKP might also offer resources for finding support groups.

Virtual Connections: Dive into online communities that cater to CKD patients for virtual support and camaraderie.

Making the Most of Support Groups

Once you've landed in a support group, here's how to maximize your experience:

Dive In: Don't hold back! Share your experiences and ask questions. Active participation enriches the experience for everyone.

Respect Fellow Members: Acknowledge that everyone's journey with CKD is unique. Offer respect and support to others, even if their experiences differ from yours.

Set Boundaries: It's okay to step back or limit your involvement if you're feeling overwhelmed.

Find Your Fit: Not all groups vibe the same way. If one group doesn't feel right, keep exploring until you find your tribe.

Virtual Connections: The World of Online Communities

Online communities offer a round-the-clock haven for CKD warriors. Here's why they're worth exploring:

24/7 Support: Whether it's day or night, online communities provide constant support, irrespective of time zones.

Anonymity: Some folks find solace in the anonymity online platforms offer, making it easier to open up about CKD-related matters.

Diverse Perspectives: You'll encounter a diverse array of individuals managing CKD from all walks of life, offering a broad spectrum of insights and experiences.

Finding Your Online Niche

There's a plethora of online platforms tailored for CKD patients. Here's where to look:

Social media: Scour platforms like Facebook or Twitter for CKD-related groups.

Forums: Many kidney organizations host forums where you can connect with fellow CKD warriors.

Disease-Specific Websites: Check out websites dedicated to CKD—they might have online communities or forums for interaction.

Navigating Online Spaces Responsibly

While online communities offer abundant support, exercising caution is key:

Trust the Pros: Remember, while others may share experiences, they aren't medical experts. Always consult your healthcare provider for medical advice.

Guard Your Privacy: Be vigilant about sharing personal details online.

Stay Skeptical: Not all information online is accurate. Approach what you read with a critical eye and seek out reliable sources for medical info.

Connecting with fellow CKD warriors can be profoundly empowering. By immersing yourself in support groups and online communities, you'll discover a sense of belonging, glean invaluable insights, and forge a network of support that bolsters your emotional well-being on this journey with CKD. In the next chapter, we'll delve into the emotional terrain of living with a chronic illness, offering strategies for managing stress, anxiety, and nurturing a positive mindset.

9.3 Advocating for Yourself: Communicating Your Needs and Goals

Living with chronic kidney disease (CKD) is a transformative experience. As you grapple with treatment decisions, adjust your daily routines, and adapt your lifestyle, effective communication with your healthcare team becomes crucial. This section aims to empower you to advocate for yourself, ensuring that your voice is heard and your needs are met throughout your CKD journey.

The Significance of Advocacy: Taking Control of Your Health

Patient advocacy involves actively participating in your healthcare journey. Here's why it's pivotal for managing CKD:

Enhanced Treatment Outcomes: By articulating your needs, preferences, and concerns, you can collaborate with your doctor to devise a treatment plan that suits your objectives and lifestyle.

Empowerment and Confidence: Advocating for yourself instills a sense of agency and enables you to make well-informed decisions regarding your health.

Strengthened Doctor-Patient Relationship: Transparent and candid communication fosters trust and cooperation between you and your doctor, paving the way for a more effective partnership in managing your CKD.

Sharpening Your Advocacy Skills: Effective Communication Techniques

Becoming an effective advocate for yourself involves refining essential communication skills:

Educate Yourself: Familiarize yourself with CKD, treatment options, and potential side effects. Armed with this knowledge, you can ask pertinent questions and actively engage in discussions with your doctor.

Clarify Your Objectives: Reflect on your priorities and desired outcomes for managing CKD. Understanding your goals enables you to articulate your needs effectively.

Prepare Thoroughly: Prior to appointments, jot down your questions and concerns. Keep a record of your medications, symptoms, and any recent health developments.

Be Direct: Communicate your needs and concerns clearly and succinctly. Don't hesitate to seek clarification or repeat information if necessary.

Express Yourself: It's perfectly acceptable to convey your emotions, whether it's apprehension, frustration, or doubt.

Open communication cultivates a supportive doctor-patient dynamic.

Cultivating a Collaborative Relationship: Engaging with Your Doctor

Your doctor is a crucial ally in your CKD journey. Here's how to nurture a collaborative rapport:

Ask Questions: Don't shy away from asking questions, regardless of their complexity. A clear comprehension of your condition empowers you to make informed decisions.

Voice Your Preferences: Share your treatment preferences and inclinations with your doctor. Let them know what aligns best with your lifestyle and comfort level.

Assertiveness with Respect: While it's vital to assert your needs, maintain a respectful demeanor. A cooperative approach yields optimal results.

Consider Second Opinions: If you harbor doubts about a treatment plan or feel your concerns are overlooked, don't hesitate to seek a second opinion from another nephrologist.

Beyond the Doctor's Office: Interacting with Other Healthcare Providers

Effective communication extends beyond your doctor. Here's how to engage with other healthcare professionals involved in your care:

Nurses: Communicate openly with nurses about any medication concerns, procedural queries, or general well-being issues.

Dietitians: Clearly convey any dietary restrictions, preferences, or challenges you encounter in adhering to a renal diet.

Social Workers: Discuss transportation, financial assistance, or emotional well-being concerns with social workers, who can offer valuable support and resources.

In Conclusion

You are the foremost authority on your body and experiences. By refining your communication skills, advocating for your needs, and fostering a collaborative partnership with your healthcare team, you can seize control of your CKD journey and navigate it with assurance and empowerment.

CHAPTER TEN

CUTTING-EDGE RESEARCH: EXPLORING NEW THERAPIES AND ADVANCEMENTS

10.1 THE SCIENCE OF HOPE: PROMISING RESEARCH FOR CKD TREATMENT

Chronic kidney disease (CKD) may be progressive, but that doesn't dim the hope for tomorrow. Researchers worldwide are delving into innovative treatment avenues and preventive measures, offering a beacon of optimism for those navigating CKD. This section plunges into the realm of ongoing CKD research, spotlighting promising areas poised to revolutionize treatment and enhance the lives of millions.

Beyond Dialysis and Transplantation: Pioneering the Future of CKD Care

While dialysis and transplantation stand as pillars in advanced CKD treatment, the scientific horizon is ever-expanding. Here are some riveting areas of research brimming with potential for the future of CKD management:

Regenerative Medicine: Envision a future where damaged kidney tissue could be rejuvenated. Scientists explore the use of stem cells to repair or replace dysfunctional kidney cells, potentially restoring kidney function.

Gene Therapy: Delving into the genetic roots of certain CKD types, researchers aim to correct genetic abnormalities through gene therapy, offering a lasting solution for some patients.

Immunosuppressive Drugs for Non-Transplant Settings: Investigating the repurposing of immunosuppressive medications beyond transplants, researchers seek to slow CKD progression by tempering the immune response that targets healthy kidney tissue.

Sodium Glucose Cotransporter-2 (SGLT2) Inhibitors: Originally devised for diabetes management, these medications show promise in retarding CKD advancement by regulating blood sugar levels and easing the burden on the kidneys.

Artificial Kidney Devices: Still in nascent stages, artificial kidney devices hold the potential for a more portable and adaptable dialysis alternative compared to conventional hemodialysis.

Precision Medicine: Customizing Treatments for Individual Needs

The future of CKD treatment likely embraces a personalized approach. Precision medicine tailors' treatment plans based on individual genetic makeup, lifestyle factors, and CKD subtype, optimizing outcomes. Imagine treatment avenues crafted to address your unique requirements, maximizing your quality of life.

Clinical Trials: Shaping Tomorrow

Clinical trials play a pivotal role in testing new treatment frontiers. By partaking in clinical trials, you not only contribute to CKD research progress but also gain access to novel treatments. Prioritize discussions with your doctor about the potential merits and risks of clinical trial participation.

Staying Abreast: Navigating the Latest Research

As CKD research continues to evolve, staying informed is key. Here's how to keep pace with the latest developments:

Reputable Organizations: Resources from esteemed entities like the National Kidney Foundation (NKF) and the American Society of Nephrology (ASN) offer accessible insights into ongoing CKD research.

Medical Journals (with caution): While medical journals unveil cutting-edge research, the jargon may pose challenges. Consult with your doctor to decipher research articles effectively.

Support Groups and Online Communities: Engage with CKD-focused support groups and online forums, where discussions often touch upon emerging research breakthroughs.

Though the road to conquering CKD is ongoing, the strides in research offer hope. While a cure for CKD may not be imminent, the scientific community's relentless pursuit promises more effective treatments and enhanced quality of life for those grappling with CKD. In the following chapter, we'll explore the realm of emotional well-being in the context of chronic illness, unraveling strategies for managing stress, coping with anxiety, and embracing resilience amidst life's challenges.

10.2 Artificial Intelligence and Precision Medicine: Personalized Solutions for the Future

Chronic kidney disease (CKD) affects millions worldwide, driving the quest for more effective and personalized treatments. Artificial intelligence (AI) is swiftly reshaping the medical landscape, offering substantial promise for precision medicine in CKD. This section delves into the dynamic fusion of AI and CKD, shedding light on how this potent technology could redefine diagnosis, treatment optimization, and ultimately, patient care.

The Influence of AI: Reshaping CKD Management

AI encompasses a suite of sophisticated algorithms and machine learning techniques adept at scrutinizing extensive medical data. Within CKD, AI offers manifold potential advantages:

Advanced Diagnosis: AI algorithms can sift through intricate medical data—like blood tests, imaging scans, and patient history—to pinpoint patterns potentially overlooked by human observation. This might lead to earlier and more accurate CKD diagnoses, facilitating prompt interventions and potentially arresting disease progression.

Risk Stratification: By analyzing patient data, AI can forecast individuals most vulnerable to CKD or its complications. Armed with this foresight, healthcare providers can enact preventive measures and tailor treatments to individual risk profiles.

Tailored Treatment Plans: By dissecting a patient's medical journey, genetic blueprint, and medication responses, AI can prescribe bespoke treatment blueprints.

This precision approach holds promise for more effective and tolerable treatment protocols.

Drug Discovery: Leveraging vast molecular databases, AI hastens drug discovery and development for CKD. This accelerated pace may yield more targeted and efficacious medications.

AI in Action: Unveiling Potential Applications

AI's impact in CKD research and management is already tangible:

Forecasting Disease Progression: AI models forecast CKD progression rates based on patient data, informing tailored treatment strategies to impede disease advancement.

Optimizing Dialysis: By analyzing dialysis machine metrics and patient vitals, AI fine-tunes dialysis settings for efficient blood filtration.

Medication Management: AI scrutinizes medical histories to pinpoint potential drug interactions and suggest personalized dosages.

Identifying CKD Subtypes: AI discerns diverse CKD subtypes from complex patient data, fostering the development of targeted treatments.

Precision Medicine: Shaping the Future of CKD Care

AI charts the course for precision medicine in CKD, where treatments aren't one-size-fits-all but rather crafted to match each patient's distinct needs and disease nuances. This tailored approach holds vast potential for enhancing treatment outcomes and life quality in CKD patients.

Challenges and Considerations: Ethical and Practical Hurdles

Despite its promise, AI in CKD care isn't without hurdles:

Data Security: Safeguarding patient data is paramount, necessitating robust data protection measures.

Algorithmic Bias: Mitigating biases in AI algorithms ensures equitable tool application.

Transparency: Understandable AI conclusions foster trust and responsible healthcare integration.

Accessibility: Ensuring universal access to AI-powered diagnostics and treatments prevents healthcare disparities.

The Road Ahead: A Collaborative Journey

Seamless integration of AI into CKD management hinges on collaborative efforts:

- Nephrologists: Doctors must adeptly utilize AI tools and interpret outputs for informed clinical decisions.

- AI Developers: User-friendly AI tools tailored to CKD needs are imperative.

- Regulatory Bodies: Clear guidelines are essential for AI tool development, validation, and implementation.

AI stands poised as a transformative force in CKD care. Yet, responsible development, transparent application, and stakeholder collaboration are essential to ensuring this technology benefits all CKD patients. In the subsequent chapter, we'll explore the emotional facets of chronic illness and delve into strategies for stress management, anxiety coping, and fostering resilience in the face of chronic conditions.

10.3 Keeping Up-to-Date: Resources for Staying Informed About CKD Research

Chronic kidney disease (CKD) is intricate and ever-changing. The realm of CKD research continuously uncovers fresh insights into disease progression, treatment avenues, and potential breakthroughs. Keeping abreast of these developments can empower you to engage in meaningful discussions with your healthcare provider, make informed choices about your care, and cultivate optimism for the future. This section furnishes you with valuable tools to stay abreast of CKD research progress.

Reputable Organizations: A Knowledge Hub

Several esteemed organizations devote themselves to CKD research, education, and advocacy, providing a trove of patient-friendly resources brimming with the latest insights:

National Kidney Foundation (NKF): A frontrunner in the battle against kidney disease, NKF's website offers exhaustive CKD information, from ongoing research endeavors to clinical trials and patient education materials.

American Society of Nephrology (ASN): Catering predominantly to healthcare professionals, ASN's website also hosts a patient education segment, furnishing resources on diverse CKD facets, including research updates.

American Kidney Fund (AKF): Dedicated to kidney disease awareness and research, AKF's website is replete with informative resources on CKD research and ongoing clinical trials.

Medical Journals: A Deeper Dive (with Caution)

While medical journals are repositories of cutting-edge research, they warrant cautious navigation:

Technical Language: Medical jargon prevalent in journals might pose comprehension challenges for those lacking a scientific background.

Study Focus: Journals primarily report research study outcomes rather than dispense tailored treatment guidance.

Consultation: Engage your doctor if you chance upon a compelling journal article to glean insights into its implications for your specific health scenario.

Support Groups and Online Communities: Sharing Knowledge and Encouragement

Forge connections with individuals grappling with CKD, as they offer invaluable support and information exchange:

Online Forums: Many kidney organizations and advocacy groups host forums facilitating information sharing, queries, and discussions on recent CKD research findings.

Social Media Groups: Scout CKD-centric groups on platforms like Facebook or Twitter, ensuring they're managed by credible entities advocating evidence-based dialogue.

Patient Blogs and Websites: Numerous patient bloggers and CKD-centric websites furnish personal anecdotes, insights, and sometimes updates on the latest research strides.

Critical Thinking: Responsible Evaluation

With a plethora of online information, exercising discernment is paramount:

Source Assessment: Scrutinize the source's credibility—does it hail from a reputable medical entity, advocacy group, or personal blog?

Publication Date: Given the dynamic nature of medical research, prioritize current information reflecting the latest insights.

Scientific Basis: Favor content supported by peer-reviewed research from credible medical journals.

Consultation: When in doubt, confer with your doctor for a professional appraisal of online findings tailored to your unique health context.

Staying abreast of CKD research is pivotal for active engagement in your healthcare journey. Leverage the provided resources judiciously, but maintain a critical stance towards online information. Always lean on your doctor to elucidate research findings and discern their applicability to your health profile. In the subsequent chapter, we'll explore the emotional facets of chronic illness, offering insights into stress management, anxiety coping, and resilience building strategies.

CHAPTER ELEVEN

LIVING WELL WITH CKD: INSPIRATIONAL STORIES OF RESILIENCE

11.1 JESSICA'S JOURNEY: FROM FEAR TO FLOURISHING WITH CKD

Chronic kidney disease (CKD) can feel like a daunting journey, marked by uncertainty and fear of what lies ahead. Jessica's experience, however, sheds light on the resilience of the human spirit and the capacity to adjust to life with a chronic illness.

Jessica, a vibrant 42-year-old accountant, was blindsided when her doctor mentioned "nephropathy" during a routine blood test. The news shook her to the core, flooding her mind with denial, fear, and countless questions about her future. What would become of her active lifestyle? Her dreams of exploring the world? Her overall health?

Jessica's fears were common among those facing a CKD diagnosis. Yet, with the unwavering support of her loved ones and a proactive mindset, she embarked on a journey of self-discovery and empowerment.

Taking Control: Embracing Education and Advocacy

Once the initial shock subsided, Jessica's determination to manage her health took center stage. She immersed herself in learning about CKD, attending informative seminars by the National Kidney Foundation (NKF) and connecting with an online support group for individuals in the early stages of CKD.

Armed with newfound knowledge, Jessica embraced dietary changes, regular exercise, and medication adherence as crucial aspects of CKD management. She prioritized open communication with her doctor, ensuring her concerns were addressed and her voice heard in her treatment plan.

Embracing Change: Establishing a New Normal

Transitioning to a new lifestyle posed its challenges for Jessica, particularly with dietary restrictions that initially left her craving her favorite salty snacks. However, with creativity and guidance from a registered dietitian, she explored a variety of flavorful and kidney-friendly recipes.

Exercise, once viewed as a chore, evolved into a source of solace and empowerment for Jessica. Joining a local walking group not only provided physical activity but also fostered connections with like-minded individuals committed to healthy living.

Strength in Numbers: The Supportive Community

The online support group became Jessica's lifeline, offering a safe space to share experiences, fears, and victories with others on similar journeys. These connections instilled a sense of belonging and optimism, as Jessica gleaned insights from fellow members' coping strategies and offered her support in return.

Beyond the virtual realm, Jessica found solace in confiding in close friends and family, educating them about CKD and its impact on her life. Their empathy and encouragement formed a robust support network that uplifted her spirits during challenging times.

Living Fully: Embracing Life with CKD

Today, Jessica thrives as a testament to resilience, refusing to let CKD define her. She continues to explore the world, adapting her travel plans to accommodate dialysis treatments if necessary. Savory and nourishing meals have become a source of joy for Jessica, who delights in discovering culinary delights that align with her dietary needs.

Jessica's journey serves as a beacon of hope, underscoring the importance of education, advocacy, and community support in navigating life with CKD. With the right resources and a positive mindset, living with CKD doesn't entail sacrificing one's dreams or quality of life.

11.2 John's Green Thumb: Cultivating Joy and Health Through Gardening

Chronic kidney disease (CKD) can certainly present challenges, but it doesn't have to overshadow your passions. John's journey illustrates how pursuing creative outlets, such as gardening, can bring joy, improve emotional well-being, and even offer health benefits for those with CKD.

John, a retired carpenter who cherished time outdoors, received his CKD diagnosis in his late 60s. Initially, shock and fear gripped him, compounded by the doctor's advice on dietary restrictions and the potential need for dialysis. For John, an active man who found solace in his garden, this news felt disheartening.

Yet, John refused to let despair take over. He decided to focus on what he could control – his attitude and environment. Recalling the doctor's guidance on maintaining a healthy weight and engaging in light physical activity, John saw an opportunity to merge his gardening passion with his new health needs.

Revamping His Garden: Beauty with Purpose

Understanding that his traditional garden wouldn't align with his dietary restrictions, John saw this as a chance to create a kidney-friendly sanctuary. He delved into research and unearthed a variety of colorful vegetables suitable for his renal diet. Herbs like basil and parsley added flavor without the potassium, while greens like lettuce and spinach provided essential nutrients within his dietary limits. John's garden blossomed into a vibrant tapestry of hues and tastes, a testament to his ingenuity and a source of nutritious produce.

Nature's Therapy: Stress Relief and Presence

Beyond providing healthy fare, gardening became a form of therapy for John. Nurturing plants, observing their growth, and immersing himself in nature offered solace and tranquility. The repetitive tasks of caring for his garden – weeding, watering, and pruning – provided a therapeutic rhythm that eased his stress, a common challenge for those with chronic illnesses.

Engrossed in his garden, John found mindfulness in the present moment. The rhythmic motions and connection with nature allowed him to momentarily escape the worries tied to CKD. Amidst the flourishing foliage, he found a sense of calm and contentment.

The Social Aspect: Sharing the Bounty

John's newfound passion for kidney-friendly gardening wasn't confined to solitude. He shared his harvest and knowledge with neighbors, some also navigating health issues. Together, they exchanged tips on cultivating low-potassium veggies, forming a supportive community that transcended gardening.

John's green haven became a symbol of resilience, inspiring others to embrace healthier lifestyles and find joy in simple pleasures.

Living with CKD, Embracing Life: Passion Enriches Living

John's journey underscores the significance of pursuing activities that bring joy, even amidst health challenges. Gardening offered him purpose, sustenance, stress relief, and community.

Remember, a CKD diagnosis need not define your life. Embrace your passions, explore new avenues, and discover inventive ways to cultivate happiness and well-being, despite the hurdles of chronic illness.

11.3 Sarah's Climb: Achieving Career Success While Managing CKD

Living with a chronic illness like CKD can undoubtedly cast a shadow over your career goals. Balancing work responsibilities with medical appointments, treatment schedules, and potential fatigue can feel like a daunting task. However, Sarah's journey serves as a beacon of hope, illustrating how you can excel in your career while effectively managing CKD.

Sarah, a driven marketing manager in her early 30s, was taken aback by her CKD diagnosis. The initial shock was quickly followed by a flood of concerns – how would this affect her demanding career? Could she maintain her high-performance level while prioritizing her health? The fear of workplace discrimination and potential limitations loomed large.

Nevertheless, Sarah refused to let fear hold her back. Instead, she took proactive steps to navigate her career path while thriving with CKD:

Transparent Communication: Building Trust with Employers

Recognizing the importance of honesty, Sarah confided in her supportive manager about her CKD diagnosis. She provided insights into the condition and its potential impact, emphasizing her dedication to her work and proactive management of her health. It's essential to carefully weigh the decision to disclose your condition to your employer, considering both the benefits and risks.

Planning and Prioritization: Optimizing Work Schedule

Sarah evaluated her workload and identified areas where adjustments could be beneficial. She discussed flexible scheduling options with her manager, exploring opportunities for remote work or flexible hours to accommodate medical appointments or treatments, if necessary.

Creating a Supportive Network at Work:

Sarah chose to confide in a few trusted colleagues about her condition. Having a supportive circle within the workplace alleviated feelings of isolation and provided a safe space to seek assistance or share concerns when needed.

Self-Care: Nurturing Success from Within

Recognizing the importance of self-care, Sarah incorporated healthy eating habits into her daily routine, ensuring access to kidney-friendly snacks and meals at work. She also made time for regular physical activity, whether it meant taking short walks during breaks or joining fitness classes during lunchtime.

Maintaining a Positive Mindset:

Despite her diagnosis, Sarah remained focused on her strengths and achievements. She refused to let CKD define her or hinder her professional growth. Her positive outlook and dedication to excellence remained unwavering.

Sarah's Triumph: Inspiring Others

Today, Sarah continues to excel in her role as a marketing manager, serving as an inspiration to those navigating careers with CKD. Her journey underscores the importance of open communication, strategic planning, and self-care. It exemplifies that with determination and the right approach, a chronic illness doesn't have to hinder professional success.

Remember: Many individuals with CKD achieve remarkable feats in their careers. By following Sarah's example, advocating for yourself, and prioritizing your well-being, you can carve out your path to professional success while effectively managing CKD. The next chapter delves into practical strategies for coping with stress, anxiety, and emotional well-being while living with CKD.

CHAPTER TWELVE

YOUR EMPOWERED FUTURE: LIVING A FULFILLING LIFE WITH CKD

12.1 EMBRACING YOUR NEW NORMAL: SETTING REALISTIC GOALS AND EXPECTATIONS

Living with chronic kidney disease (CKD) can feel like a significant life upheaval. It's entirely normal to ride a rollercoaster of emotions, from denial and frustration to fear and uncertainty. However, amidst this emotional whirlwind, taking control and establishing achievable goals is key to navigating your new reality and reclaiming a sense of empowerment over your health.

In this chapter, we'll deep into the importance of setting realistic goals and expectations when living with CKD. We'll discuss strategies for adapting, maintaining a positive mindset, and ultimately, thriving despite the obstacles.

Assessing Your Starting Point: Understanding Your Needs

The first step in setting realistic goals is assessing your current situation:

Severity of CKD: Understanding your CKD stage helps determine the adjustments you may need to make.

Current lifestyle: Evaluate your habits, from diet and exercise to daily activities, and identify areas for potential changes.

Emotional well-being: Acknowledge your feelings and anxieties. Prioritizing goals that support your mental health is crucial.

SMART Goals: A Blueprint for Success

Utilizing the SMART framework ensures that your goals are attainable and contribute to your overall well-being:

Specific: Clearly define your objectives. For instance, instead of "eat healthier," aim for "include three servings of vegetables in my daily meals."

Measurable: Quantify your goals to track progress and celebrate achievements.

Attainable: Set challenges that push you but remain within reach considering your limitations and health status.

Relevant: Ensure your goals align with your health objectives and contribute to your well-being.

Time-bound: Establish deadlines to create urgency and maintain motivation.

Breaking Big Goals into Manageable Steps

Overwhelming goals can be daunting, so break them down into smaller, more manageable tasks. For instance, if you aim to increase physical activity, start with short walks three times a week and gradually ramp up intensity or duration as you progress.

Prioritizing Self-Care: Nurturing Your Journey

Self-care is vital for effectively managing CKD. Focus on:

Healthy Eating: Work with a dietitian to develop a personalized kidney-friendly meal plan.

Regular Exercise: Incorporate physical activity like walking or swimming to boost energy and mood.

Stress Management: Practice relaxation techniques like meditation or deep breathing to alleviate stress.

Quality Sleep: Aim for sufficient rest each night to support overall well-being.

Embracing Flexibility: Adjusting Expectations

Living with CKD requires adaptability. There will be good and bad days, and unforeseen challenges may arise. Stay flexible and celebrate every small victory along the way.

Building a Support System: Sharing Your Journey

Don't face CKD alone. Surround yourself with supportive friends, family, and healthcare professionals. Joining a support group can provide invaluable emotional support and connect you with others on a similar journey.

Remember: Setting realistic goals empowers you to manage CKD effectively. By focusing on progress and embracing flexibility, you can embrace your new reality and lead a fulfilling life despite the challenges. The next chapter will explore practical strategies for managing stress, anxiety, and emotional well-being while living with CKD.

12.2 Celebrating Milestones: Recognizing Your Progress and Achievements

Living with chronic kidney disease (CKD) can often feel like a relentless challenge, with a focus on managing limitations and overcoming obstacles. However, it's crucial to celebrate your progress and achievements along the way to stay motivated and foster a sense of accomplishment.

This chapter emphasizes the importance of recognizing your victories, no matter how small, on your journey with CKD.

Shifting Your Perspective: From Limitations to Progress

It's easy to feel overwhelmed by the restrictions that come with CKD. However, focusing solely on these limitations can be discouraging. Instead, cultivate a growth mindset. Acknowledge and celebrate your achievements, regardless of their size.

Did you manage to incorporate an extra serving of vegetables into your diet this week? Celebrate it! Did you walk for 30 minutes without feeling overly fatigued? That's a victory! By recognizing your progress, you reinforce positive behavior changes and boost your confidence in managing CKD.

Tracking Your Journey: Keeping a Progress Journal

A progress journal is a powerful tool for recognizing your achievements. Write down your goals, both big and small, and track your progress toward them. This allows you to visually see how far you've come, which can be incredibly motivating, especially during setbacks.

Celebrating Milestones, Big and Small

Here are some examples of milestones worth celebrating on your CKD journey:

Maintaining Healthy Blood Pressure: Keeping your blood pressure within the recommended range is crucial for CKD management. Achieving this through medication or lifestyle changes is a significant victory.

Sticking to Your Diet: Dietary modifications are a cornerstone of CKD management. Celebrate the days or weeks when you follow your kidney-friendly meal plan.

Incorporating Regular Exercise: Starting and maintaining a physical activity routine can be challenging. Celebrate milestones like completing your first exercise session or increasing the duration or intensity of your workouts.

Managing Stress Effectively: Developing healthy coping mechanisms for stress is a major achievement. Celebrate mastering relaxation techniques or finding healthy outlets for releasing stress.

Openly Discussing CKD with Loved Ones: Opening up about your diagnosis can be difficult, but having a supportive network is vital. Celebrate open and honest communication with family and friends.

Sharing Your Victories: Building a Supportive Community

Don't underestimate the power of sharing your victories with your support system. Tell your family and friends about your accomplishments, no matter how small they may seem. Join an online support group for people with CKD and celebrate successes together.

Sharing your journey with others who understand can be incredibly motivating and provide valuable support during challenging times.

Rewarding Yourself: Recognizing Your Efforts

Celebrating your achievements goes beyond a mental pat on the back. Consider rewarding yourself for reaching milestones. This positive reinforcement strengthens your commitment to your goals and reinforces healthy behaviors.

Note: Living with CKD is a journey, not a destination. Celebrate every step you take toward effectively managing your condition and improving your overall well-being. Recognizing your progress, big and small, fuels your motivation and empowers you to navigate the challenges of CKD with a positive and resilient spirit.

12.3 Living with Purpose: Building a Life You Love Despite CKD

Chronic kidney disease (CKD) can feel like a thief, stealing your sense of control and disrupting the life you once envisioned. But CKD doesn't have to define your existence. You can still lead a fulfilling, purposeful life filled with passion, joy, and meaningful connections. This chapter explores strategies for building a life you love despite the challenges of CKD.

Finding Your Why: What Ignites Your Passion?

Living with purpose starts with introspection. Ask yourself:

What are my values? What truly matters to you? Is it spending time with loved ones, helping others, pursuing a creative passion, or continually learning new things?

What brings me joy? Which activities or experiences fill your life with happiness and fulfillment?

What are my strengths and talents? What are you good at? How can you leverage your skills to make a positive impact?

Identifying your purpose provides direction and motivation, especially when navigating the challenges of CKD. Maybe it's spending more quality time with family, volunteering for a cause you care about, or finally pursuing that creative hobby you've always put off.

Embracing New Possibilities: Reframing Limitations as Opportunities

CKD might impose some limitations, but it doesn't have to extinguish your dreams. Reframe limitations as opportunities to explore new avenues. Can't participate in high-impact sports anymore? Maybe it's time to discover the joy of yoga or swimming. Dietary restrictions can be an opportunity to explore new and delicious kidney-friendly recipes.

Focusing on What You Can Control

A diagnosis of CKD can feel overwhelming, with a seemingly endless list of things you can't control. However, focusing on what you can control empowers you to take charge of your health and well-being. This includes:

Diet: Making healthy food choices is a powerful tool for managing CKD symptoms.

Exercise: Regular physical activity, even in modified forms, boosts energy levels and improves overall health.

Stress Management: Developing healthy coping mechanisms for stress can significantly influence your well-being.

Sleep Hygiene: Prioritizing adequate sleep is crucial for physical and mental health.

Medical Adherence: Following your doctor's recommendations and treatment plans is vital for managing CKD effectively.

Building a Supportive Network: Enlisting Your Tribe

Living with CKD is easier with a strong support system by your side. This network can include:

Family and Friends: Share your diagnosis and treatment plan with loved ones. Their understanding and support can be invaluable.

Healthcare Team: Your doctor, nephrologist, and registered dietitian are your partners in managing CKD. Open communication and collaboration are key.

Support Groups: Connecting with others who understand the challenges of CKD can provide emotional support, share coping mechanisms, and foster a sense of belonging.

Living in the Present Moment: Cultivating Gratitude

Living with a chronic illness can make it easy to dwell on future or past uncertainties. However, focusing on the present moment and cultivating gratitude for the good things in your life can significantly improve your outlook. Practice mindfulness techniques like meditation or deep breathing to ground yourself in the present. Express gratitude for good health days, supportive relationships, and the little joys in life.

Living with CKD, Not Defined by It

CKD is a part of your life, but it doesn't have to be your entire story. You can build a fulfilling and purposeful life filled with passion, joy, and meaningful connections. By focusing on what you can control, embracing new possibilities, and cultivating a supportive network, you can thrive despite the challenges.

CONCLUSION

Chronic kidney disease (CKD) can feel like an unwelcome detour on your life's journey. The initial diagnosis might bring fear, uncertainty, and a whirlwind of "what ifs." But with the knowledge and tools from this book, you can navigate this new path and build a fulfilling life, CKD and all.

As you embark on this journey, remember that everyone's experience with CKD is unique. There will be good days and bad days, moments of frustration, and times of triumph. Here are some real-life situations to illustrate the points covered in this book:

Picture Sarah, the marketing manager from Chapter 11.3. She thrived in her fast-paced career before her CKD diagnosis. Initially worried about disclosing her condition, she chose to communicate openly with her understanding manager. Together, they explored flexible work arrangements to accommodate doctor's appointments and dialysis if needed. Sharing her diagnosis with trusted colleagues created a supportive network within the office. By prioritizing self-care, including healthy meal planning and regular exercise, Sarah maintained her energy levels and thrived in her demanding role.

Think about John, the green thumb from Chapter 11.2. After his diagnosis, John's initial despair turned into a determination to find joy despite the limitations. He embraced kidney-friendly gardening, transforming his space into a haven of vibrant vegetables and herbs. Nurturing his plants became a form of stress relief and mindfulness. John's newfound passion wasn't just about healthy food; it fostered a sense of purpose and social connection as he shared his harvest and knowledge with neighbors.

Recall Jessica's story from Chapter 11.1. The fear and uncertainty that gripped her after the diagnosis gradually transformed into a proactive approach to managing her CKD. Jessica devoured educational resources, joined a support group, and actively participated in treatment plan discussions with her doctor. She embraced dietary modifications and discovered a world of flavorful kidney-friendly recipes. Exercise, once a chore, became a source of empowerment and stress relief. Jessica's story exemplifies the power of education, self-advocacy, and finding a supportive community.

These examples show how individuals with CKD can chart their course to a fulfilling life. Remember the key takeaways from this book:

Embrace education: Empower yourself with knowledge about CKD, treatment options, and healthy lifestyle choices.

Focus on what you can control: Diet, exercise, stress management, and medication adherence are powerful tools in managing CKD.

Build a support network: Surround yourself with loved ones, healthcare professionals, and support groups who understand your journey.

Celebrate your victories: Recognize your progress, big or small, to stay motivated and maintain a positive outlook.

Live in the present moment: Cultivate gratitude for the good things in your life and find ways to embrace each day.

Living with CKD doesn't mean sacrificing your dreams or passions. With the right approach, you can navigate the challenges, embrace new possibilities, and create a life filled with purpose, joy, and connection. This book has been your companion on the first leg of this journey. Now it's your turn to take charge, embrace your new normal, and continue writing your remarkable story.

"Thanks for reading! If you enjoyed this book or found it useful, I'd be very grateful if you'd post a short review on Amazon. Your support really does make a difference and I read all the reviews personally so I can get your feedback and make this book even better.